MEDITE

MADE EASY

Quick, Simple and Delicious Recipes To Prevent Disease, Lose Weight, and Live Better

Simon Matthews

MEDITERRANEAN DIET MADE EASY

Quick, Simple and Delicious Recipes To Prevent Disease, Lose Weight, and Live Better

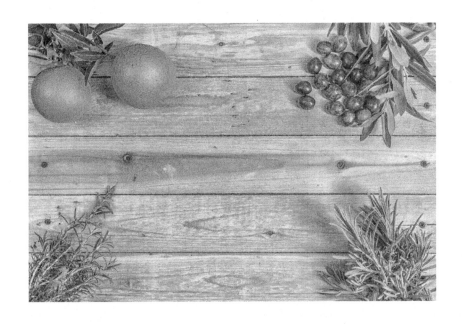

TABLE OF CONTENT

CHAPTER 1

UNDERSTANDING THE MEDITERRANEAN DIET

What is the Mediterranean diet?

In order to start talking about the Mediterranean diet it is important to know that the word diet derives from the Latin word diaeta, which comes from the Greek "diaita", which means "way of life", which can also be interpreted as "lifestyle", therefore, the Mediterranean diet is the Mediterranean lifestyle, that is, the way the Mediterranean people live.

The Mediterranean diet is nothing more than a diet based on the dietary patterns of various countries bordering or influenced by the Mediterranean Sea. Even though they had different cultures, it was observed by researcher Ancel Keys (1904-2004) in the 50's to 60's, in a research entitled "Study of Seven Countries" - where the dietary patterns of the following countries were studied: Japan, Finland, Netherlands, United States, former Yugoslavia, Italy and Greece - that these countries had a common diet, mainly due to the soil and climate of these regions, creating a typical fauna and flora, bringing a diet composed of the same foods. This research was one of the guidelines that brought the relationship between diet and heart disease, where it was observed that although these countries had a high-fat diet, the level of people living in these regions (such as southern Italy and

Greece) had high life expectancy rates and low levels of heart disease, which has led many researchers and food experts to rate this diet as one of the healthiest in the world! Researchers at the University of Barcelona have come to the conclusion that this food program could prevent about 30% of heart attacks that lead to death, as well as prevent strokes and cardiovascular disease.

This diet consists of a diet based on fresh in natural foods, taking from the diet any processed foods. Thus, various chemical additives are eliminated from the diet routine, in addition to the excess salt and sugar present in most processed foods. Foods such as fish (tilapia, sardines and salmon), fruits and vegetables, good fats (moderate consumption of extra virgin olive oil), nuts, whole grains, dairy products, water and moderate consumption of red wine are part of the menu of this diet and should be consumed daily, some more moderately, others more often. Certain foods, such as red meat and chicken, for example, can be eaten sporadically as long as they are never fried but roasted, grilled or cooked; It is recommended that the main intake of animal protein comes from fish, which should be eaten three to four servings per week.

In addition to numerous health benefits, the Mediterranean diet is a diet that helps change the lifestyle of its supporters, as it naturally improves metabolism and favors weight control, even eating higher calorie foods than other diets. Weight loss is noticed in the first weeks of the diet, which satisfies its fans to continue to have a balanced and balanced diet. Regular exercise should also be associated with this diet, ensuring faster and more satisfactory results.

The History Of The Mediterranean Diet

There were several historical periods that had great influences on the Mediterranean diet.

The popular trade at the time (A.C.) among the great civilizations, allowed for the expansion of Mediterranean food products. Regions such as Mesopotamia, Aegean, Phenicia, and later Carthage exported olive trees, figs, grapes, and almonds, and brought Asian peppers and spices to the West, and it was these diverse settlements that also introduced wheat, rye, oats, citrus fruits, mutton and goats for the Mediterranean countries.

Already the Romans modified the commodities by colonization, where all the territory conquered at the time should cultivate olive and grape trees. That was how they marked the limits of their power. They imposed wheat in areas such as Turkey, Egypt, Greece, Sicily, Andalusia, and Languedoc, where there were cultivated peas, beans, lentils, chickpeas, and leafy greens, all brought from eastern areas of the Roman Empire.

In turn, the Arabs spread citrus fruits all over the Mediterranean area while the Byzantines and especially the

Ottomans had a major influence on culinary practices in the 12th and 13th centuries. However, sugar cane and rice were introduced during the Crusades. The beginning of contact with China in 1298 allowed the importation of new products such as pasta and fruits such as cucumber and pulses. Some references say that the Mediterranean diet was formed in two essential periods: Classical Antiquity and Roman Empire, in Classical Antiquity, international trade began to develop and this allowed the Roman Empire to modify dietary habits at the time strongly. The Arabs, on the other hand, protected diversity and disseminated their agronomic and technical knowledge. During the discoveries of the Americas, some products introduced via Spain and Portugal have become raw materials in the Mediterranean area, such as corn, potatoes, tomatoes, sweet peppers, calabash and chocolate. Finally, in the last colonization made around the 19th and 20th centuries, they brought Maghreb soft wheat, lentils, corn, tomatoes, salad, artichoke, asparagus, chestnuts and acorns.

As already mentioned, the Mediterranean diet was popularly known thanks to the North American Dr Ancel Keys through the study known as "Study of the Seven Countries". In 1941, Keys was asked to develop a US Army ration suitable for soldiers to carry with them in combat. This food was produced through hard crackers, dry sausages, chocolate bars and hard candies. When the army began mass-producing the packages, they marked them with the letter K in honour of Dr Keys, and thus the K ration was born. During World War II, Keys served as Secretary of War's special assistant and noted that the deaths heart disease dropped dramatically in countries where supplies were low during the war, and it was around this time that he began to look for a connection. The concept of the Mediterranean diet was born through the Study of Seven Countries, begun by Keys in 1950, which will be discussed in more detail in the next section of this book.

In short, the Mediterranean diet is based on practical dietary patterns in countries bordering the Mediterranean Sea, such as Greece, Southern Italy, France and Spain. These patterns were identified from 1940 to 1950.

The Science Behind The Mediterranean Diet

The first clinical evidence that found the health benefits of the Mediterranean diet came from the Lyon study called the "Lyon Diet Heart Study," which followed 605 patients who suffered myocardial infarction. After four years, these patients adhered to a Mediterranean-style diet and achieved a 55% reduction in the risk of death and a 50 to 70% reduction in the risk of developing new cardiac complications.

However, it was Ancel Keys, previously mentioned, the researcher responsible for publicizing this diet, following a study he conducted in several Mediterranean countries. The study was conducted for over 15 years and was named "Coronary Heart Disease in Seven Countries", popularly known as "The Study of Seven Countries". This study continues to have a great influence even today, and many others have been developed or inspired by this study that was primordial for the knowledge of the Mediterranean Diet. In this study, it was found that the increase in coronary disease onset was directly related to the increase in fat consumption. However, there was a significant exception observed in Mediterranean countries, which even given the high fat intake, the occurrence of cases of myocardial infarction was much smaller compared to other countries. It was this relationship that piqued the interest of Ancel Keys, who concluded that this was due to the type of food practised in these countries.

The study was conducted with the participation of nearly 13,000 men (thirteen thousand) aged 40 to 59 years in seven countries, namely: Yugoslavia, Italy, Greece, Finland, the Netherlands, the United States and Japan. The main variables taken into account were: smoking, weight, physical activity, resting heart rate, electrocardiogram, lung capacity, blood cholesterol levels, blood pressure and diet. With these parameters in hand, Keys and his team built mathematical models to determine, as far as possible, their relationship to the risk of coronary heart disease.

After the initial data collection, the variables were compared again 5 to 10 years later, between 1958 and 1970, resulting in a series of conclusions, later published in 1980 in the book "Seven Countries: A Multivariate Analysis of Death and Coronary Heart Disease. Mortality and coronary artery disease"). He came to the following conclusion:

As for lifestyle, the percentage of saturated fat present in the diet proved to be the best predictor of heart disease, where it was found that the higher the consumption of saturated fat, the higher the risk.

The most important of the quantifiable and proven physiological variables by examination was cholesterol, in addition to hypertension (the second most important risk factor for heart attacks).

Although Keys' original work was considered one of the pioneering studies leading the Mediterranean diet to be known worldwide as the supposed paradigm of healthy eating, it received several criticisms that questioned the way the researcher initially exposed the "fat hypothesis" and about your final remarks. One of the criticisms generated around his study was that the basis of his theories was created from a graph, which showed the almost perfect correlation between the amount of fat in the diet and mortality from heart disease. This graph was contested by two authors of the time, namely: J. Yerushalmy and H. Hilleboe, who questioned the fact that the research was based on only seven countries, and there were 22 countries that could have participated in this important research. Had the 22 countries been chosen instead of just 7, this correlation would not be as perfect as the proposal and conclusions would be much different.

Although there is controversy about the studies by Keys, many others are still made based on this study considered primordial for the knowledge of the Mediterranean diet. In addition to this study, Keys published a book titled "Eat well and stay well" that became a bestseller and gave the Keys couple a cover in Time magazine in the January issue of 1961. This book provided guides for the preparation and culinary use of various foods, and where and how to purchase them. It was with this book that the media eventually coined and spread the well-known term: the Mediterranean diet.

Recently, the Mediterranean diet has been included since 2010 in the list of Intangible Cultural Heritage of Humanity of UNESCO. However, the main reason for being included is due to concepts related to knowledge, practices, traditions, culinary use, cultivation, harvesting, fishing, conservation, elaboration, preparation and consumption. It was these aspects that earned him this mention as a heritage and not exclusively because it is considered beneficial for health - this figure among one of the reasons for this mention, but is not the most important.

CHAPTER 2

LIVING HEALTHY WITH THE MEDITERRANEAN DIET

When it comes to diet, many people think of missing out on the food they love so much. However, diet is not something that should be viewed as boring or restrictive. The diet itself is nothing more than something that can be modified according to the nutritional needs, goals and/or dietary restrictions that each of us may have. Already a balanced or balanced diet consists of the set of foods, amounts, frequency of feeding, along with fluid intake and regular exercise, which help achieve the goals required in each diet.

The Mediterranean diet is a diet that has a great dietary pattern, providing a great diversity of foods, being a diet rich in fats, fruits, legumes, cereals, spices and herbs, vegetables, vegetables, eating wine in meals, fish and fruits. From the sea. Even though it is high in fat, this diet is considered one of the healthiest eating patterns today.

The Benefits Of The Mediterranean Diet

Based on research and studies, it has been proven the numerous benefits that the Mediterranean diet can provide to its fan, being one of the few diets with scientific proof of its benefits. Some benefits of the Mediterranean diet are Energy: Because it is a diet that has a high consumption of whole cereals, these with low glycemic index and vegetable oils that have good amounts of fatty acids - such as omega 3 and omega 6 - these Foods act as energy sources, giving us more energy to face everyday life.

Regulated bowel: Since there is the regular consumption of vegetables and fruits, and legumes and being these foods sources of fibre, help the proper functioning of the intestine.

Cardiovascular disease prevention: Intake of omega 3 and omega 6 rich foods contributes to the increase in good cholesterol, known as HDL (High-Density Lipoprotein) being found in olive oil, fish and almonds; and in decreasing triglycerides and bad cholesterol, known as LDL (Low-Density Lipoprotein) thus preventing cardiovascular disease.

Lowers Cholesterol: There are good cholesterol and bad cholesterol. LDL brings cholesterol to cells and facilitates their deposition of fat in the vessels and is considered as bad cholesterol, while HDL promotes the removal of excess cholesterol, including arterial plaques, which is why it is called good cholesterol. Foods like olive oil, fish, almonds and some pulses are high in good cholesterol, whereas processed foods and fried foods are high in bad cholesterol. As this diet is banned from eating these foods, its effectiveness is greater in reducing it and consequently prevents the development of various heart diseases.

Increased Muscle Mass: Foods Considered Builders Like fish, eggs and poultry, they are present in this diet and have large amounts of amino acids, which are responsible for the repair and formation of muscle mass.

Strengthens the Immune System: Rich in foods high in amino acids, such as honey, ginger, almonds, garlic and collard greens; They are responsible for maintaining the immune system and help in preventing numerous diseases. Studies show that people who eat this diet besides having a long and healthy life, hardly get flu or sick from diseases that we get for low immunity.

Principles, Advantages And Disadvantages Of The Mediterranean Diet.

At the very beginning, it should be mentioned that the Mediterranean diet is not a way to lose extra weight or fight obesity. It's a healthy lifestyle, a diet that allows us to keep our body in the best condition. The Mediterranean diet is a nutrition pattern inspired by foods consumed by the inhabitants of the Mediterranean coastal areas. Many studies have shown that people living in this area live longer than the average European population and enjoy better health. The genesis of the diet is exactly known and falls in the 1950s and 1960s. It began exactly in 1948 when the Greek government turned to the Rockefeller Foundation for nutritional tests among the inhabitants of Crete and nearby villages. Studies have shown that fats make up approx. 38% of energy consumed per day, but these are healthy fats - primarily olive oil. At that time, Cretans also consumed a lot of coarse-grained products, fish, vegetables and fruit. The daily habits of the inhabitants of the coastal villages also included drinking dry red wine with each meal. Ancel Keys took care of the Mediterranean diet in the following years. He linked the low incidence of cardiovascular disease, cancer and other diets - dependent diseases with the consumption of products typical of the Mediterranean diet. Inspired by his insight, he gathered a team of doctors and began to study seven countries, the so-called Seven Country Study, which confirmed that the Mediterranean diet is very healthy and reduces the risk of cardiovascular disease in adults. Wine for health - history, artistry of production and types of this aromatic drink, which means - truth is in wine, but is there anything more to it? read more Mediterranean diet - principles The basic source of carbohydrates in the Mediterranean diet are pasta dishes. They are consumed in huge quantities with tomato sauce, cheese and olive oil. Sometimes, only on special occasions, pieces of meat or seafood are added to them. Farmers could not afford to afford such luxuries. Most meals were accompanied by a bite of self-made cereal bread. Once or twice a week, the Cretans ate dinner, instead of pasta, meat or sea fish. Fresh fruit was eaten daily for dessert. Rules of the Mediterranean diet: The diet must be very abundant in products of plant origin, we are talking here not only about fresh fruit and vegetables, this includes cereals, bread, legumes, nuts, seeds and potatoes. These products are a good source of energy, complex sugars and fibre. The right amount of plant-based products protected people from vitamin and mineral deficiencies. High fibre intake lowered cholesterol and protected against many gastrointestinal diseases. Food should be as little processed as possible, in the 1960s farmers did not have access to processed food products; usually, the products came from their own farms or were bought in nearby villages from farmers and sellers. Thanks to such cooperation, people built their economy and also had access to varied crops depending on latitude and season. Fresh fruit in the Mediterranean diet has always been served as a dessert after a hearty dinner. The Mediterranean diet does not avoid the consumption of simple sugars; it is recommended to consume honey or sweets with high sugar content 2-3 times a week. Olive oil is the main source of fat, it is added to pasta, salads, and dry bread is dipped in it. The classic Mediterranean diet contains 8% energy from NKT (Saturated Fat), 13% energy from JNKT (Monounsaturated Fat) and 9% energy from WNTK (Polyunsaturated Fat). Dairy products in the Mediterranean diet are primarily yoghurt and white cheese: mozzarella and feta, less often parmesan cheese. They were consumed in small quantities. Several times a week, you can afford fish and poultry, these are lean meats, they are eaten primarily due to a large amount of full-value protein present in them. You can eat 2 to 4 eggs a week (including baked goods and other products prepared from them). Red meat is consumed in the Mediterranean diet several times a month. The wine drunk with each meal is dry and red. In addition to all the above principles of the Mediterranean diet, it is also important to exercise moderate physical effort every day. The peasants had good health because they worked on their farms. Agriculture in the 1960s was not as well developed as it is today, not every family could afford agricultural machinery, most of them had to cultivate their own land or with the help of utility animals. If you want to see a transparent graphic model of the Mediterranean diet, I recommend that you familiarize yourself with the official Willet's food pyramid from 1995. cholesterol Nothing reduces cholesterol as effectively as a diet! The hypolipemic diet is an ally of our health. Especially for people struggling with the problem of high blood cholesterol. read more Mediterranean diet - advantages One can talk a lot about the benefits of the Mediterranean diet. There are many arguments that support its introduction into our lives. It is said to have anti-cancer effects. It is associated with the presence of beta carotene, vitamin E, vitamin C and selenium with a strong antioxidant effect. The Mediterranean diet also has a lot of fibre - it binds excess bile acids, reduces the passage time of the gastrointestinal tract, inhibits the procancerogenic effect of short-chain fatty acids. By reducing the passage time of the nutrient content, the risk of colorectal cancer is significantly reduced. The amount of plant-derived products consumed also correlates with the incidence of cardiovascular disease. This effect can also be associated with high fibre intake, and more specifically, its soluble fraction. A dose of 2-3 g of soluble fibre fraction in the diet reduces the concentration of total cholesterol in the blood, protecting us from developing atherosclerosis. It also reduces blood pressure and blood glucose. Consuming a large amount of fruit and vegetables provides a solid dose of potassium for the diet - studies in the United States have found a link between potassium intake and reducing stroke. Olive oil is the main source of fat in the Mediterranean diet. Fats consumed in the Mediterranean diet are primarily vegetable fats, mainly olive oil. Its use in the diet increases the healthy fraction of HDL cholesterol, while it does not affect the harmful LDL fraction - reduces the risk of developing ischemic heart disease. An interesting fact about olive oil is the fact that regardless of the amount of its consumption, there is no research proving its harmfulness. The consumption of dairy products such as natural yoghurt and white cheese brings a lot of benefits in the Mediterranean diet. Milk was not often consumed in the 1960s, because few poor farmers could afford refrigeration equipment in which they could be stored. Calcium contained in cheese and yoghurt is very well absorbed; it is well absorbed. Reduces the risk of osteoporosis in adults in old years, while significantly increasing their quality of life. Another benefit of dairy products is that calcium also has blood pressure-lowering properties - while reducing the risk of hypertension and other cardiovascular diseases. It is also worth mentioning that the substances contained in fermented dairy products have a beneficial effect on the intestinal bacterial flora and their work. Fish, poultry and eggs bring full-value animal protein to the diet, it is rich in essential amino acids, without which our body quickly deteriorates in health. They also contain cholesterol necessary for the production of salts and bile acids, as well as for the synthesis of certain vitamins and hormones. Oily marine fish is the main source of n-3 fatty acids in the Mediterranean diet - responsible for normalizing blood pressure and breaking up potential blood clots that can lead to heart attacks. It is interesting that in the Mediterranean diet, alcohol is an integral part of all meals. With each meal, the inhabitants of Crete consumed 1-2 glasses of dry red wine. It was not as strong wine as the one we get in stores today; it was diluted with water in a 1: 1 ratio with meals. Screening tests for a wide group of Crete residents have shown that the presence of alcohol in the diet reduces the risk of atrial fibrillation by 30%. Red wine is also indicated due to the presence of phenolic substances in it. The most important of them is resveratrol, which is an active substance on the LDL cholesterol fraction - thus reducing the possibility of atherosclerotic changes and free radical oxidation. Mediterranean diet - disadvantages The Mediterranean diet has a few disadvantages. It is planned in a fairly transparent and clear way. It can be used as a daily diet for the rest of our lives. It provides us with vitality and strength every day. In addition, we can enjoy good health. You can use the Mediterranean diet as a way to lose weight. In my opinion, it is only then that we can talk about its disadvantages. Weight loss on a Mediterranean diet is not fast; optimal results are achieved if we lose 3-4 kg within 2 months of a strictly controlled diet and moderate exercise. Comparing to other weight-loss diets, the Mediterranean-Mediterranean effects wait quite a long time, and this can demotivate some people. Another big disadvantage is the fact of counting calories - to lose weight, you should write a diet for the number of calories lower than our total metabolism by about 500-1000 kcal. And such a diet should be used for a minimum of three months. The problem arises when the reduced amount of calories needs to be divided into 4-5 meals a day, remembering the right proportions of fats, proteins and carbohydrates. It requires good organization and great self-control. Despite several disadvantages of the Mediterranean diet, its advantages definitely speak for its use. We then achieve long-term health results. We eat healthily and feel good. Applying this style of nutrition does not cost us much, and in addition, drinking small amounts of wine every day will allow us to relax after a hard day, stress, school or work ... I encourage you all to try this diet! You will certainly like it, and you will not want any more.

Planning Your Mediterranean Diet

The mediterranean diet is a characteristic diet of people living in countries bordering the Mediterranean Sea as its name implies, being a diet based on the dietary pattern of those countries.

Many carbohydrates they consume derive from vegetables and legumes. The consumption of bread, for example, is more moderate and even when consumed, is made with wheat, which over the years had minor changes, given the weather and other factors. This wheat has a lower amount of gluten, which makes it less resistant during digestion, whereas the wheat we consume here in Brazil, besides being different, has a higher amount of gluten, which makes it more resistant. Given this example, it is a fact that even if we adopt this diet, its effectiveness will not be the same as these countries can, because of the differences in cultivation, region, place and climate that these foods are grown, such as wheat.

The fish found in these regions have higher amounts of omega 3 than those found here. In addition to the regions that certain favourite foods, the way they cook and treat the food enhances the nutrients and minerals of each food, thus increasing its effectiveness. That said, can we do the Mediterranean diet without being in Mediterranean countries? Yes, you can adopt this diet with the foods found in our country, respecting the main rules stipulated by this diet.

To have good planning, it is important to know all the foods that are allowed and those that are prohibited. Fruit consumption can be adapted to seasonal fruits, which will allow us plenty of options.

10 Tips To Succeed

Changing your diet or lifestyle is no easy task, especially for those who are used to eating everything and how much they want. Having a healthy and balanced diet is much more beneficial to our lives not only for the present but for our future as well, because, in addition to making us lose weight, it improves our health and ensures us healthy ageing by protecting us from disease and ensuring longer longevity. Following are some tips on how to succeed in our Mediterranean diet.

Tip 1: Avoid radical and very restrictive diets

If you go on a diet that deprives you of some food you know you can't go without, it tends not to be as successful as it should be, as it will always have the risk that you will fall into temptation and eat what is forbidden. After all, we always have the thing that "what's forbidden tastes better." Prefer diets that fit your tastes. Look for a nutritionist to help you build a healthy and enjoyable menu.

Tip 2: Replace processed foods with natural foods

This is one of the most valuable tips you can follow as it will ensure you greater success in your diet. Processed products tend to be more caloric, high in sodium and sugars, and super fatty. In between your meals, invest in healthy snacks that contain a larger combination of different food groups, such as vegetables, nuts, cereals, fibre and protein.

Tip 3: Eat carbs for breakfast

Carbohydrates are great sources of energy and help us cope with everyday life. They should be eaten preferably in the morning as you will have all day to spend them. Invest in whole-grain bread or fibre-rich breakfast cereals.

Tip 4: Escape the fried foods

Fried foods tend to have a higher amount of saturated fat and large amounts of calories. Avoid eating meat, chicken or fried fish. Give preference to grilled and roasted foods, whereas in vegetables prefer steamed or sauteed.

Tip 5: Replace ready seasoning with herbs and spices

Ready-made seasonings contain lots of sodium and chemical additives, as well as altering the natural flavour of the food. Replace with fresh herbs and spices, which in addition to adding flavour to your food, are rich sources of vitamins and can be grown and grown in small gardens indoors, which besides being much healthier encourages children to eat better and better. in a healthier way.

Tip 6: Eat less and more often

Decreasing portion sizes is a fundamental part of any diet because portion sizes of each food are important factors that will or will not guarantee the success of your diet. Eating too much, even if you eat the foods allowed in the diet, has the opposite effects. Eat smaller portions, but at smaller intervals, such as every 3 hours. In addition to leaving us satiated longer, this will increase our metabolism, which will ensure us lose weight. Skipping meals or eating at long intervals makes us eat more food than necessary, which contributes to weight gain.

Tip 7: Make a list and go to the full belly supermarket

Having a list of the foods we need to buy will only pay attention to the items on the list, making us avoid buying prohibited products in our diet, such as processed foods. Just be mindful of buying the products listed and escape the temptations. Another valuable shopping time tip is to go to the supermarket with a full belly after a meal. When we are hungry, even if focused on healthy eating, we are tempted to eat other foods that are available to us at that time. Going hungry for a candy showcase, for example, can become a torment because the chance of falling into temptation is much greater.

Tip 8: Chew each food well and escape distractions during meals

Chewing food calmly and several times helps in the process of digestion of food and makes us understand that we are already satisfied. Eating in a hurry tends to make us eat more because as we take 2-3 bites, our brain thinks we only eat 1, so eating 1 bite and chewing it very well, will make us eat less, and that ends up reflecting on the control — our weight. Avoiding mealtime distractions is also an important tip because when we are distracted, we end up eating more than necessary; try eating your meal in front of the television one day and the next eating with the television off, you will realize that you had eaten more when you were watching your favourite show than when you were focused on your meal because you will not realize how much you ate for being distracted.

Tip 9: Drink plenty of fluids

Staying hydrated is also super important for any diet, because when we are dehydrated our body tends to retain fluids and leave us swollen, so always have a bottle of water at your disposal. The volume of water intake varies according to various factors such as routine and exercise; however, this intake should be around 1.8L to 2L of water for sedentary people, and 3L for more active people, athletes and other extreme sports practitioners tend to take up to 5L of water a day.

Tip 10: Regular exercise practice

Regular exercise is an important aspect of the Mediterranean diet. Maintaining a light walking or running routine is of great importance to the success of who is practicing this diet. In addition to giving us greater physical endurance, helps increase metabolism, blood circulation prevents various cardiovascular diseases, and has the effect of leaving us strong and fit.

CHAPTER 3

EATING ACCORDING TO THE MEDITERRANEAN DIET

In the traditional diet, carbohydrate consumption is 5 to 9 servings daily, while in the Mediterranean diet consumption is not limited. However, their intake is made in a conscious and balanced way, being divided better during meals. Fruit and vegetable consumption is recommended in both diets, as these are sources of vitamins and nutrients. The ideal is their consumption in natural (raw), but if you want to make them cooked it is ideal to be steamed because this way they preserve more nutrients and vitamins while enhancing the natural taste of these foods.

Another weight difference between the Mediterranean diet and the traditional diet is the consumption of fats such as olive oil. In the Mediterranean diet, its consumption is daily and can be used even in recipes that are part of breakfast. In the case of the traditional diet, its consumption is avoided, being considered a villain of cholesterol. Note: It is important to note that although the Mediterranean diet includes the use of olive oil in almost every meal, its use is controlled and its calories included in the calculation of the given meal, i.e. if a tablespoon of olive oil has 100kcal and your meal should be around 300kcal, assuming a brochette if you have olive oil as one of your ingredients, the sum of the others cannot exceed 200kcal.

In the traditional diet, meat, chicken and fish are consumed on a regular basis and are consumed more often than in the Mediterranean diet, which prefers fish in small portions weekly. Seafood is also included in the Mediterranean diet, while in ordinary diets, their consumption is more sporadic.

Sweets are different on both diets. In the case of the Mediterranean diet, sweets are sweetened with honey instead of traditional sugars, whether refined, demerara or brown. In traditional diets, we have opted for the consumption of refined sugar, which is changing over time, as people have focused more on their health and cut down on foods considered harmful to health such as sugar. An interesting thing about sweets from Mediterranean countries is that they tend to be salty, with a mixture of cereals, nuts, almonds and dried fruits. Brazilian sweets, for example, tend to have a higher sugar concentration, such as chocolates, cakes and pies.

Another important difference found in the Mediterranean diet compared to the traditional diet is the consumption of wine at meals. For the people of the countries bordering the Mediterranean Sea, wine is not only present during meals, but also part of them. Its consumption is moderate, but it is frequent. In the traditional diet, alcohol intake is moderate and not included in meals, and of course, exceptions at special events and dates.

As we can see in the two pyramids, there are considerable differences between them, the traditional food pyramid is based on carbohydrates such as bread, rice, cereals, pasta and roots, while in the Mediterranean diet food pyramid the base of the pyramid is the practice of exercises physicists. It is on this basis that the whole diet is assembled, and is therefore considered one of the healthiest in the world today.

What You Can Eat

Dietary guidelines are divided into daily, weekly and occasional frequency. Below we will see what you can eat and how often you eat according to your specific group.

Throughout the day: water, infusions, broths; In daily meals: cereals, vegetables, fruits, vegetables, olive oil; Daily: spices, herbs, garlic, onions, olives, nuts, seeds, dairy products, wine; Weekly: fish, white meat, eggs, pulses; Occasionally: red meat, processed meat, potatoes; Weekly on special occasions: sweets.

Shopping basket in the Mediterranean diet

Many questions may arise when it comes to what to put in the grocery basket. In this topic, I will cover what you can buy and what to avoid on your visit to the grocery store.

1. Avoid shelves: It sounds simple, but it is very important. Avoid products found on supermarket shelves. In general, most of them are processed products and/or contain some chemical additive, which is not good for our diet.

2. Abuse fresh fish: Look for a fish shop in your city and avoid buying fish from supermarkets. As the turnover of these products may not be frequent, it is best to buy from specific fishmongers. Abuse salmon, tuna, sardines, tilapia, but prepare them roasted or grilled, never fried! The intake should be around four servings per week.

3. Avoid red meat: Red meat is not prohibited on this diet, but given its history and lifestyle of the people of the Mediterranean, eating red meat is virtually none. The best known and most consumed protein comes from fish and seafood, but of course, we can adapt to our lifestyle; and for those who do not give up a good

steak, the tip is to give preference to lean cuts such as filet mignon, for example. Another tip is to restrict your consumption to one serving per week. This goes for chicken cuts too. Your preparation (either for meat or chicken) should preferably be grilled or roasted.

4. Fruits and Vegetables: In order to maintain the required nutritional properties, portions of fruits and vegetables should be ingested daily.

Vegetables should be steamed. One ingredient regularly found in various forms is tomatoes. It is present in salads, sauces and garnishes, is rich in lycopene and should be guaranteed presence at meals. Salads should be explored and assembled to taste. They should be frequent at both lunch and dinner. Fruits can replace desserts, complement lunch and be part of the snack between the main meals, such as the morning and afternoon snacks.

5. Good Fats: Extra virgin olive oil is a great example of good fat present in this diet. Rich in antioxidants that are beneficial to heart health, extra virgin olive oil can be used to season and prepare salads and fish, however, their consumption should be moderate and included in the meal calorie calculations. According to a study by scientists from various European

universities and published in the Diabetes Care of the American Diabetes Association, it has been shown by volunteer imaging that taking two tablespoons of this powerful oil daily is enough to absorb what The foods have better and keep the body in shape.

6. Chestnuts: If you don't find it in your local supermarket, look for little shops that sell natural products and be sure to abuse the nuts, walnuts and almonds. They give you a feeling of satiety and avoid overeating during meals and are rich in cholesterol-controlling substances. They can be eaten with fruit at mealtimes as a snack, or included with meals as part of the ingredients.

7. Whole Grains: Invest in Whole Foods, Vegetable Proteins such as lentils, beans and chickpeas should be part of the daily eating routine. The substitution of white rice for brown rice and macaroni for brown rice. Also, replace the daily french bread for whole-grain bread. These are small changes that cause numerous health benefits and help us regulate the intestines.

8. Dairy products: Yogurt, milk and cheese are part of the Mediterranean diet menu and should be consumed daily, watch out for low-fat products. In the case of cheese, preferably white. In the case of milk, prefer skimmed and nonfat or nonfat yoghurt.

9. Wine: Wine is also part of the menu and complements this diet rich in nutrients, minerals and vitamins. For those who do not drink alcohol, the substitution of wine for whole grape juice can be done, but its benefits will not be the same. Wine is rich in polyphenols and resveratrol, substances that protect the heart. In addition, they have components that act as antioxidants which help in reducing bad cholesterol and increases good cholesterol. Obviously, your consumption should be moderate. Excessive consumption of alcohol leads to an increase in triglyceride levels, thus increasing the vascular risk. Therefore, always keep in mind that wine is a complement to the meal and not something that can be abused during the day today. One tip is to consume 100ml or half a glass of red wine during dinner.

10. Frozen Foods: Escape from ready and frozen dishes. They are usually rich in preservatives, chemical additives and are very greasy. Prefer to prepare food always on time, so you ensure a higher concentration of food nutrients.

11. Avoid Buying Too Much: Foods like fruits and vegetables, leaves and vegetables should be bought weekly, if possible in small quantities so that they are not left in the fridge, preserving

food is essential so that they can keep its nutritional characteristics. Check the best way to keep each food group, either inside or outside the refrigerator, and always separate spoiled and rotten food from good and healthy so that there is no contamination.

Eating out

One thing is for sure; there's nothing better than hanging out with friends, family or loved ones to share a meal, isn't it? And when we are on a diet, this activity that is so pleasing to us makes us uneasy. Will we be able to keep the diet even eating out? There are some tips that can help you stick to your diet without depriving yourself of the pleasure of hanging out with our friends.

Drinking-Water Before Meals: Having a glass of water at least half an hour before meals help to dilate our stomach, leaving us more satiated, and consequently we eat less.

Ask first: If your outing with friends is to a ready-made restaurant, ask first of all. Opt for healthier, fewer calorie dishes, asking first you will not be influenced by that friend who ordered a cheese-bacon accompanied by chips with a lot of maturity and bacon.

Eating in the self serve: If your way out is to a restaurant where you can help yourself, help yourself and sit down, wait for everyone who is accompanying you to help you and sit down. Wait for everyone to start your meal. This act is not just a matter of education, but it will prevent you from finishing first and ending up repeating. That way everyone will finish their meals at the same time.

How to behave at work-related meals: Being under pressure during a work meeting is no longer pleasant, and when it comes to having to eat, things seem to get worse. Eating anxiously or under pressure makes us eat more than necessary, so if you are in this situation, ask for a dish where you need to chew a lot, such as a dish that has meat or salad. Avoid dishes that are quick to chew.

Meals with people who don't care about healthy eating: you know that friend who doesn't care to have a healthy meal eating? Yeah, I'm not saying you should ignore it and block it from your life, however when it comes to healthy eating, if you don't want to be influenced by poor diet choices, eat healthy snacks or satiety fruits before going out to eat or drink. So when they arrive at the restaurant or bar, you will no longer be hungry, and you can eat in a conscious way.

Willpower and focus: Changing the diet is not an easy task, especially if the person is not in the mood to do so. Many end up choosing diets, either by medical indication or some dietary restriction, and this is often not welcomed. Changing the feed should be gradually and without that pressure. Replacing those calorie meals with healthier dishes that are palatable will help a lot in this new trajectory. With willpower and focus, you can control yourself on a meal that you have to eat out without skipping the diet.

How to assemble the plate

When we stand in front of the buffet many questions arise as to how to set up the dish, which foods to put, which to avoid, how much of each food to put on the plate and how many calories it should have, and of course, countless other questions that may arise. Below I have listed some tips on how to assemble your plate in a healthy way without escaping your diet.

First, take that basic look at the buffet before serving, so you can know what you like and dislike, what you can and can't eat.

Ideally, the dish should average 300 to 400 calories, not to mention dessert and drink.

The food should be in the centre, leaving the edges visible.

The salad should occupy 50% of the dish, which should consist of vegetables (escape the mayonnaise salads and specks), avoid the industrialized sauces and prefer to season with olive oil and vinegar; Pickled foods such as corn, peas, palm hearts and olives are high in sodium and should, therefore, be consumed in small quantities.

In its other half, the dish should contain brown rice plus beans (about 2 tbsp each). The protein is meat, which can be red or chicken. Look for low-fat meat, if it is even better fish, give preference to grilled and avoid roasts and fried (the portion should be equivalent to the palm of your hand not exceeding 100g of meat).

For dessert, prefer fruit, fruit salads or desserts with low-fat yoghurt.

For the drink, escape from the industrialized juices and sodas. Prefer natural juices, coconut water or even a tea.

DAY 1

Breakfast

1 slice light brown bread + 1 teaspoon ricotta cream

1 cup unsweetened green tea

Morning snack

200 ml of pineapple juice with watercress leaves

Lunch

1 plate of dark green salad leaves + 1 teaspoon extra virgin olive oil + balsamic vinegar

2 tablespoons rice 7 bowls of cereal + ½ cooked lentil shell

1 sardine fillet

200 ml whole grape juice

Afternoon snack

1 bowl of fruit salad + 1 tablespoon light granola

Dinner

1 plate of watercress salad with cherry tomatoes

2 tablespoons brown rice with carrot

1 fillet of fresh herbs

Supper

1 cup mint tea + 5 units pistachios

DAY 2

Breakfast

1 unit light whole meal toast + 1 teaspoon natural unsweetened fruit jelly

200 ml peach unsweetened soy juice

Morning snack

1 lime orange + 1 Brazil nut

Lunch

1 plate raw coleslaw + 1 tablespoon extra virgin olive oil

2 tablespoons cooked white beans

1 cup steamed broccoli, cauliflower and asparagus

1 Grilled Chicken Breast Fillet

200 ml whole grape juice

Afternoon snack

3 black plums + 2 apricots

Dinner

1 Plate of American Lettuce Salad with Radish

2 tablespoons Greek rice

1 crab cone

Supper

1 cup jasmine tea + 2 cashews

DAY 3

Breakfast

1 slice light brown bread + 1 teaspoon light cottage cheese

1 cup unsweetened red tea

Morning snack

1 cereal bar with nuts

Lunch

1 plate of escarole salad with ½ chopped mango + 1 tablespoon extra virgin olive oil

2 tbsp brown rice

2 tablespoons fresh peas

1 salmon fillet with passion fruit sauce

200 ml whole grape juice

Afternoon snack

200 ml of coconut water

Dinner

1 plate (dessert) of grilled vegetables

2 sardine fillets

100 ml dry red wine

Supper

1 cup lemon balm tea + 1 Brazil nut

DAY 4

Breakfast

1 slice whole-wheat bread + 1 slice minas cheese + 1 tomato slice

+ 1 tablespoon extra virgin olive oil + fine herbs and salt to taste

½ papaya papaya

200ml sweetened lemon juice with 1 tsp brown sugar

Morning snack

6 strawberries + 1 walnut

Lunch

1 plate of dark green leafy salad + ½ grated carrot + cherry tomatoes + 1 teaspoon extra virgin olive oil

2 tbsp brown rice + 2 tbsp french fries

1 piece of baked cod with buttered potatoes

200 ml whole grape juice

Afternoon snack

1 fruit and cheese skewer

Dinner

1 plate of salad leaves + 2 tomato slices + radish + 1 teaspoon olive oil

1 flat plate of fettuccine with seafood and herbal oil

100 ml dry red wine

Supper

1 cup chamomile tea + 2 almonds

DAY 5

Breakfast

1 mashed silver banana + 1 teaspoon ground cinnamon + 1 tbsp oatmeal

1 cup unsweetened black coffee

Morning snack

1 gala apple

Lunch

1 plate of leafy salad with broccoli and cauliflower + 1 teaspoon extra virgin olive oil

2 tbsp brown rice + 2 tbsp french fries

1 roast croaker fillet

200 ml whole grape juice

Afternoon snack

2 slices of white cheese

1 thin slice of watermelon

Dinner

1 plate of salad leaves + 1 tablespoon extra virgin olive oil

1 flat plate of whole-grain tuna noodles

100 ml dry red wine

Supper

1 cup fennel tea + 2 almonds

DAY 6

Breakfast

Papaya half papaya + 1 Brazil nut + 1 almond

1 cup of pineapple peel

Morning snack

1 pear

Lunch

1 plate of lettuce leaves salad + 3 chopped strawberries

+ grated carrots

5 tablespoons shrimp risotto

200 ml whole grape juice

Afternoon snack

1 cup of passion fruit juice + 1 tablespoon of flaxseed

Dinner

1 plate of salad leaves + 1 tsp extra virgin olive oil + 1 tsp balsamic vinegar

100 g buffalo mozzarella + 3 chopped walnuts

100 ml dry red wine

Supper

1 cup of chamomile tea + 1 nut

DAY 7

Breakfast

1 jar of nonfat yoghurt + 3 units dried apricot + 1 tbsp honey

1 cup unsweetened red tea

Morning snack

½ avocado + 1 tbsp granola + 1 tbsp honey to sweeten

Lunch

1 plate of warm mediterranean salad

5 tablespoons shrimp risotto

200 ml whole grape juice

Afternoon snack

1 cereal bar and dried fruits

Dinner

1 plate of salad leaves + 1 tsp extra virgin olive oil + 1 tsp balsamic vinegar

1 plate (dessert) of carrot cream, orange, honey and cilantro

100 ml dry red wine

Supper

1 cup fennel tea + 2 almonds

CHAPTER 4

MEDITERRANEAN DIET AND SLIMMING

The Mediterranean diet is not a typical slimming diet. Of course, it can be adapted to reduction menus, reducing caloric content; however, the basis of the Mediterranean diet as a lifestyle lies in good relations with food and eating to satisfy hunger (but no more without bingeing!).

In the US News & World Report ranking, it ranks 14 among slimming diets and 28 among diets that allow you to lose weight quickly. Eating in a Mediterranean way should also not be afraid of gaining weight despite the presence of fat in the diet. It is now well known that the consumption of sugar rather than fat is the most responsible for excess weight - all the more at its healthy sources. Several studies have shown that you can lose weight healthily with a Mediterranean diet.

However, the scientific position in this case supported by the analysis of 21 studies on weight loss using the Mediterranean diet says that specialists still do not know whether this diet is slimming and whether it protects against overweight and obesity. In 2008, the New England Journal of Medicine published the results of a study of 322 medium obese adults. They were divided into 3 groups using different diets: low-fat with limited calories,

Mediterranean with limited calories, and low-carb without caloric restrictions.

After two years, the average weight loss in the Mediterranean diet group was 4.4 kg, on a low-fat diet - 2.9 kg, and on a low-carb diet - 4.6 kg.

RULES FOR HEALTHY AND SAFE WEIGHT LOSS

The only way to lose weight is to limit food, change your diet, and increase physical activity. Slimming aids in the form of teas or slimming tablets will do nothing without your effort. Regardless of whether you want to lose a few or a dozen kilos, the principles of healthy, safe weight loss are the same. The main difference is the time to reach the goal.

Above all, healthy slimming requires patience. New, wonderful slimming diets appear every season, but let's be honest - there are no magic dishes or food sets that will help you lose weight without sacrifice. The only thing that results is a reduction in the amount of calories consumed. You've probably tried more than one boring diet, to no avail. Now we offer you a healthy weight loss program that will help you overweight once and for all and finally enjoy your dream figure.

1. Take care of a varied menu

The monotonous menu promotes food shortages, and this adversely affects metabolism. Therefore, when limiting calories, remember about important nutrients and take care of a varied menu. Every day, eat products from various groups that provide the body with the right amount of protein, carbohydrates, fats, vitamins, and minerals.

From cereal products, you should choose those from full milling (including thick cereal, whole wheat bread, brown rice, oatmeal), because they are a source of complex carbohydrates, which are absorbed more slowly and gradually release energy. In addition, they stimulate metabolism and provide B vitamins and minerals necessary during slimming. Complex carbohydrates are also vegetables that cannot be missed, taking care of a nice figure. They can appear in the form of salads for lunch, as a vegetable for dinner or as an addition to a morning sandwich. The censored ones are simple carbohydrates (contained, among others, in white bread, cookies, jams), which, in addition to a large dose of calories, give energy only for a short time.

A good source of wholesome protein is milk and its products (choose lean!) And white meat (e.g., chicken, turkey) and fish. It is also worth eating leguminous vegetables (beans, chickpeas, peas), which are rich in vegetable protein. Protein should be in every meal because it is the main building block of our tissues; in addition, it gives a longer feeling of satiety after a meal and speeds up metabolism.

Choose vegetable fats (rapeseed oil, olive oil, sunflower seeds) from fats and significantly reduce animal ones by replacing them with leaner substitutes, e.g., cream - yogurt, butter - high-grade margarine in a mug, pork - poultry, fatty sea fish (e.g., salmon, herring). To reduce the amount of fat in dishes, give up frying for baking, stewing or steaming.

2. Eat regularly

Another principle of healthy weight loss is regularity - it's best to eat 4-5 small meals a day, then your body will burn calories easier. If you skip one meal, it will make the next one bigger, or other snacks will come along. Therefore, after a mandatory breakfast before leaving home at work, do not just sit on the water, eat a healthy lunch, lunch - so you will have less appetite in the evening. Try to eat at fixed times, and eat the last light meal at least 2-3 hours before going to bed, because feasting just before bedtime results in extra kilos. During meals, focus on what you have on your plate, chew slowly (the brain gets a message about satisfying hunger only after 20 minutes from the start of the meal), finish eating with a slight hunger.

3. Remember about fiber

Fiber is extremely important in slimming because it absorbs water and swells in the stomach, giving you a feeling of satiety. At the same time, it improves bowel function and helps cleanse the body of toxic waste products. Whole grains, vegetables, and fruit contain the most fiber. The latter should be chosen carefully because some (e.g., grapes, bananas) contain a lot of sugar and thus calories. A lot of fiber and fewer calories include in raspberries, apples, currants, gooseberries, strawberries, kiwi, while pineapple, grapefruit, and papaya have a slimming effect.

4. Get hydrated and give up alcohol

Drink approx. 2 liters of fluid daily. The best choices are water, green tea (slightly stimulates metabolism), fruit, and herbal teas without sugar because they do not contain calories. Drink them regularly throughout the day, without waiting for you to feel thirsty, and drink a glass of water before meals - so you'll eat less. Avoid sweetened carbonated drinks and lots of fruit juices because they have a lot of sugar. You can reach for vegetable juices. Give up alcohol during your diet as it contains only empty calories. Most of them are in drinks, cocktails, and also in beer. Occasionally you may be tempted by a dry red wine (rich in antioxidants).

5. Introduce natural fat burners to your diet

Adding spicy spices to your dishes - pepper, chili, ginger, horseradish, or mustard - is a good way to boost your metabolism. They stimulate the production of heat (thermogenesis) in the body and help you lose weight. Record holders among natural thermogenic are chili peppers - they increase calorie burning by up to 20%. In contrast, gingerol contained in ginger accelerates the burning of fat accumulated on the stomach and internal organs. Remember to limit salt because it retains water in the body. According to WHO recommendations, you can consume up to 6g of salt per day (a teaspoon), but you only need to play for the body to work properly.

It will be useful to you

How many calories do you need per day?

a mentally working woman - 2300 kcal

a woman who works physically - 2800 kcal

a man working mentally - 2400 kcal

men working hard physically - 4000 kcal

6. Choose an activity that will please you

You do not have to go to the fitness club every day, but try to exercise 2-3 times a week for about 45 minutes, because only 30 minutes after starting the workout, your body begins to burn fat. Aerobic exercises, e.g., Nordic walking, running, cycling, swimming, are the best. You can also exercise, dance, visit the gym - it's important to do what you like. The effort should be varied because then he shapes different parts of the figure. However, the benefit of movement is not only a firm body but also better metabolism, because a kilo of muscles burns three times more calories than a kilo of fat. Exercise also reduces the levels of weight-promoting hormones such as cortisol by secreting stress-relieving endorphins, and increases the production of fat-burning hormones, including testosterone, growth hormone,

7. Get enough sleep - short sleep promotes weight gain

Studies show that sleeping people increase levels of ghrelin (hunger hormone) too short, and leptin (satiety hormone) decreases - that is, when you sleep, you are more hungry, and it is harder to satisfy your appetite. In addition, a study at the University of Chicago shows that healthy people deprived of deep, slow-wave sleep for three days (the phase in which the highest amount of growth hormone is released) decreases sugar processing capacity by 23% (they become insulin resistant). However, too long sleep is also not beneficial for the figure, because, according to research by Canadian scientists, people sleeping less than 7 hours or longer than 9 hours weigh an average of 2 kg more and have a larger waist size than those who sleep 8 hours on day.

8. Tame stress because its excess slows down metabolism

Excessive stress can upset the hormonal balance in the body. According to dr. Scott Isaacs, a specialist in the field of hormones, author of the book "The Leptin Boost Diet," stress contributes to leptin resistance, reduced body sensitivity to insulin, decreased estrogen levels in women, and testosterone in men decreased growth hormone, increased cortisol, thyroid disorders. And each of these changes slows down metabolism. Research from American scientists shows that chronic stress also increases the secretion of hunger hormone, which explains the irresistible desire for something sweet in a stressful situation. Find your way to stress. Sometimes, to get rid of bad emotions, you need to ride a bike 30 km, break a plate (or even a few), dance all night, or cry in the sleeve of a friend. In times of crisis, reach for raw vegetables, e.g., cut into sticks a carrot or kohlrabi. But if you feel that you are not able to cope with stress and you have a tendency to "eat" problems, go to a psychologist - you will gain proven methods of fighting tension.

9. Do not be discouraged when the slimming pace is too slow

At the beginning, it loses weight faster, but after a few weeks, the declines may stop. The body adapts to less energy and new mass. Then it is necessary to tighten the diet (caloric content is reduced by 200 kcal) and increase physical effort (e.g., from 1 to 2 times a week). This is a new stimulus for the body, which will again increase "turnover."

10. Don't worry if you break the diet from time to time

Do you fancy a cake, ice cream, or pork chops? Sometimes you can afford it. But remember that small offenses do not become the rule, because they ruin the whole plan. If you eat extra calories, don't blame yourself for lack of discipline, just reduce your next meal a bit or get on your bike. Many nutritionists even say that the so-called meal cheat, or "cheated" meal on a diet once a week even helps to lose weight.

Mediterranean Diet And Diabetes

Mediterranean diet reduces the risk of developing metabolic syndrome - one of the risk factors for diabetes.

An analysis of 9 studies, covering 122,000 adults, showed that compliance with Mediterranean diet guidelines reduces the risk of developing type 2 diabetes by 19%.

Another 2014 study published in the Annals of Internal Medicine concerned 3,500 seniors who had not yet developed type 2 diabetes. After 4 years, it was found that people on a low-fat diet are at greater risk of diabetes than those on a Mediterranean diet.

One of the analyzes of 9 studies involving a total of nearly 1,200 people with type 2 diabetes, using different diets, showed that people on a Mediterranean diet improved glycemic control, lowered body weight, cholesterol, and blood pressure.

Diabetic diet in accordance with the principles of healthy nutrition

Diabetic diet, in addition to drugs that lower blood sugar, is the basis for the treatment of diabetes. Diabetes does not have to give up good cuisine. Diabetic diet can also be tasty and varied; just follow a few rules. Check what the diabetic diet is, what you can eat, and which products are contraindicated.

The diabetic diet is not at all complicated, and diabetes is taking a toll on it. It is estimated that more than 2 million people suffer from it in Poland, for example. For about 1 million the disease is asymptomatic. Type 2 diabetes is the most common; it attacks 90% of the time. It is most common for people struggling with obesity after 40 years of age.

Diabetic diet and various types of diabetes

A diabetic diet is an essential element in the treatment of all types of diabetes. Among the disorders of carbohydrate metabolism, several varieties of the disease are distinguished:

- type 1 diabetes in which the pancreatic beta cells stop producing insulin; appears in children;
- type 2 diabetes, in which the tissues become insulin-insensitive and the pancreas "burns" at some point as a result of increased insulin production; is mainly the result of a poor diet;
- LADA diabetes - autoimmune diabetes of adults usually appearing after 30 years of age; is a milder type 1 diabetes;
- MODY diabetes - diabetes mellitus of young adults usually diagnosed between 20 and 30 years of age with a course similar to type 2 diabetes, but without insulin resistance;
- Gestational diabetes - hyperglycaemic conditions appearing in pregnant and healthy women before pregnancy.

Regardless of the type of diabetes, the main diet goals, and nutritional recommendations remain the same. Dietary management focuses primarily on glycemic control.

People who are overweight and obese must use menus that enable them to lose excess weight. For the early stages of type 2 diabetes and gestational diabetes, a well-composed diet is enough to keep your blood glucose steady without taking medication.

The most demanding diet is type 1 diabetes, where you need to balance your insulin intake to the amount of carbohydrates and proteins you consume. Gestational diabetes emphasizes strict control of carbohydrate intake at each meal. The least calculation requires a diet in type 2 diabetes.

Diabetic diet, or what?

The official recommendations of the diabetic diet have, for a long time, been based on guidelines limiting fat in the diet and recommending carbohydrates with a glycemic index below 55 as the main source of energy in the menu. The Polish Diabetes Association in guidelines for 2017 still recommends that 45 percent energy in the diet came from carbohydrates (and even 60 percent, if they are high-fiber products), which with a standard diet of 2000 kcal, is as much as 250 g and is associated with eating carbohydrates in virtually every meal.

This type of diet recommended for many years did not bring the expected results. It did not allow a satisfactory way to control blood glucose and reduce diabetes-related parameters, such as glucose fasting or glycated hemoglobin HbA1c.

Currently, the best diet in diabetes is a low-carbohydrate diet with increased fat content. Its effectiveness is confirmed by large, reliable scientific research, as well as practice in a dietetic office.

In their publication, they refer to the lack of effects of a low-fat diet with a low glycemic index and the side effects of drugs used in type 2 diabetes. They call on the medical community to reject the traditional approach that did not allow to control the epidemic of diabetes and to recommend patients a low carbohydrate diet. However, there is one good low carbohydrate diet recommended for everyone.

It should be remembered that carbohydrates do not provide more than 30 percent — energy in the diet. You should not be afraid of good quality fat, which does not contribute to weight gain and is not a significant risk factor for cardiovascular disease, which is also confirmed by new scientific studies. When planning meals, you can rely on the paleo diet fashionable in recent years, but also introduce the right grain products. This nutritional approach allows people with type 2 diabetes to even give up drug treatment altogether, and people with type 1 diabetes to reduce their insulin intake.

Diabetic diet – rules

The basic principle of a diabetic diet is to limit carbohydrates in meals. This applies to both simple carbohydrates (all sweets, fruits, juices, drinks) and complex ones (cereal, rice, pasta, bread, potatoes). The daily menu should not contain more than 100 - 150 g. Proponents of very low carbohydrate diets recommend consumption below 50 g per day.

The choice of carbohydrates is very individual and should be adjusted so that the sick person can easily control glycemia. Carbohydrates should come from good sources: sourdough rye bread, thick groats, quinoa. Fruits are best limited to 1 serving per day, as they are sources of simple sugars. Shop sweets, sweetened jams, juices, and drinks, as well as sweeteners, are not recommended. Various sweeteners affect glycemia even though they do not contain sugar. Meals should be eaten 4-5 times a day at more or less constant times. If nocturnal hypoglycemia occurs, a sixth meal is introduced before bedtime.

A protein-fat breakfast is very important in the treatment of diabetes. Shortly after waking up, the reaction to the sugars consumed is the largest, the easiest is hyperglycemia, and a carbohydrate-free breakfast allows good glycemic control from the morning throughout the day. Studies show that people consuming protein-fat breakfasts make better food choices and are less likely to hunger during the day. Practice in the diet room shows that the use of BT breakfast helps a lot in reducing fasting glucose. Another important meal is dinner, which in turn should contain a portion of carbohydrates to maintain stable blood sugar levels at night.

Fiber is very important in the diabetic diet. It slows down the absorption of sugar from food and has a beneficial effect on bowel function. It's best if the fiber comes from vegetables.

Fat in diets with reduced carbohydrate content is 30-50 percent. It should come from natural sources, e.g., butter, olive oil. Foods rich in fat include avocados, nuts, pumpkin and sunflower seeds, fatty sea fish, coconut milk. In particular, the very unhealthy trans fats present in hard margarine and fryers should be avoided.

Note:

Meals in the diet should be as natural as possible, prepared with fresh products. They should have a low glycemic load, which is due to the presence of protein and fat. Cereal additives should not be overcooked. Deep frying is not recommended. Avoid highly processed foods, sweets, sugary drinks, ready meals, and junk food. Alcohol should appear in moderate amounts. The basis of the diet should be vegetables. Do not binge. It is worth controlling the size of portions consumed and body weight. Physical activity is always indicated.

Diabetic diet - scientifically proven effectiveness

Limiting carbohydrate intake has the greatest impact on lowering blood glucose levels.

Glycemic control is the primary goal of treating both type 1 and type 2 diabetes. It is well known that among the macronutrients of foods, carbohydrates contribute the most to increase blood glucose levels. It should, therefore, be obvious that reducing your carbohydrate intake will help you lower your glycemia effectively. Hussain and colleagues examined 102 diabetics and 261 healthy people for 24 weeks. All study participants were divided into 2 groups, one of which was on a typical low-calorie diet and the other on a very low carbohydrate diet (VLCKD). After 24 weeks, the diabetic group on the VLCKD diet had fasting glucose levels lower by 18 mg / dL compared to the group on the low-calorie diet. On average, glycated hemoglobin was 1.5 mg / dL lower in the VLCKD group than in the low-calorie group.

A low carbohydrate diet is very effective for weight loss

The authors of the publication "Dietary carbohydrate restriction as the first approach in diabetes management: Critical review and evidence base" even use the statement that there is no more effective slimming diet than a diet with a very low carbohydrate content. This confirms one study in which 52 people took part. 26 had a very low carbohydrate diet (40g carbohydrates per day) for 3 months, and another 26 a low-fat diet. In each group, there were 13 people with diabetes and 13 healthy people. After 3 months, an average weight loss of 6.9 kg was recorded in the low carbohydrate group, and in the low-fat group - by 2.1 kg. Many long-term studies show that low-fat diets with a low glycemic index are not a tool for long-term weight loss. Low carbohydrate diets seem much better.

Carbohydrate-restricted diets allow for better glycemic control even without weight loss.

The recommendations for diabetics often emphasize weight loss conducive to glycemic control. Low carbohydrate diets appear to lower blood glucose levels even if body weight remains the same. If carbohydrates provide 20-30% of energy during the day during 10 weeks, you can see a decrease in fasting glucose even above 50 mg / dL, as well as a decrease in fluctuations in blood glucose levels during the day.

Total fats and saturated fats contained in food have no relation to the risk of cardiovascular disease. Diet hypothesis: assuming that the consumption of fat in food promotes atherosclerosis, heart attacks, and other cardiovascular diseases was established in the mid-twentieth century. Since then, many credible large studies have been published that have clearly indicated that the replacement of polyunsaturated or carbohydrate saturated fat has no effect on reducing the risk of cardiovascular disease. You should not be afraid of higher fat content in low carbohydrate diets.

Limiting carbohydrates in your diet is the best way to lower your TG levels and increase HDL cholesterol in your blood.

This is not a cereal-based diet rich in products with a low GI, but a low-carbohydrate diet is most effective in reducing parameters indicative of metabolic syndrome. One study involved 84 obese people with type 2 diabetes. They compared the effects of a VLCKD diet (20 g carbohydrates per day) and low IG on body weight, glycated hemoglobin, fasting glucose, total cholesterol, LDL cholesterol, and HDL cholesterol triglycerides. Slightly better results on the VLCKD diet were achieved for weight loss and fasting glucose; however, the level of glycated hemoglobin was 10% lower compared to the group on a low IG diet, and the level of TG - by nearly 50%. Carbohydrate restriction also contributed to a 6% increase in HDL while no changes on a low IG diet.

People with type 2 diabetes on a low carbohydrate diet limit and, in some cases, completely give up medication. People with type 1 diabetes take lower doses of insulin.

Reducing carbohydrates allows you to control your blood glucose much easier, which is why it is possible to reduce the dose of drugs and insulin. For example, in a study of 11 people on a low-carbohydrate diet without caloric restriction, 5 reduced or completely discontinued one of the diabetic drugs, and 2 could quit all drugs. In the group of 13 people on a low GI diet, only 1 person reduced the dose of the drug. In another study, 17 out of 21 people with type 2 diabetes reduced or discontinued pharmacological agents.

Mediterranean Diet And Cancer

It is currently believed that compliance with the Mediterranean diet guidelines can prevent colorectal cancer in 25% of cases, breast cancer in 15-20%, prostate, endometrial, and pancreas in 10-15%. Greek EPIC analysis of 22,000 adults over a 4-year Mediterranean diet regimen showed a 24% decrease in cancer mortality.

An observation of 350,000 Americans lasting 5 years and conducted by the National Institute of Health showed a 17% decrease in cancer mortality in men and 12% in women if some recommendations of the Mediterranean diet were followed.

Based on the analysis of the global EPIC population, it is concluded that compliance with only 2 of the basic dietary recommendations reduces the risk of developing cancer and/or dying from cancer by 6%.

What to eat so you don't get cancer? An inadequate diet can largely contribute to cancer. Which products have anti-cancer effects and accelerate the growth of cancer cells? Incorrect diet causes about 35-40% of cancers - specialists estimate. Excess kilos and obesity increase the risk of developing mouth cancer, throat cancer, larynx cancer, esophageal cancer, stomach cancer, pancreatic cancer, liver cancer, colorectal cancer, kidney cancer, prostate cancer, breast cancer, ovarian cancer, and uterine cancer.

Obesity and cancer

Women whose BMI is too high have higher than normal body estrogen synthesis. This increases your predisposition to developing ovarian and endometrial cancer. Obese women who did not give birth, had their first menstruation early, and menopause went late, more often they have breast cancer.

Men with too high body weight are more likely to develop prostate cancer, stomach, and colorectal cancer. Unfortunately, we are still unaware of the importance of daily food choices and caring for proper weight for cancer prevention. And from clinical studies, it is clear that people with a genetic predisposition to developing cancer, thanks to a proper diet, can protect themselves against cancer. Tumor formation is a long-term process. The factors that accumulate their creation are the environment, weight control, and the provision of nutrients and minerals at the appropriate level. One of these ingredients is selenium - an essential trace element that must be supplied in food.

Studies of people who got cancer of the large intestine show that in most cases in their bodies, the level of selenium was far too low. However, it cannot be said unequivocally that low levels of selenium are a carcinogen, as detailed studies in this direction have not yet been done.

Low levels of selenium in the body should, however, be a factor that will draw attention to the need for additional research, change of diet, supplementation of missing elements, etc., because in Poland, for example, people with low selenium levels develop colorectal cancer 10 times more often than people with appropriate concentration of this trace element.

The best sources of selenium:

dried porcini mushrooms, wheat, Brown rice, oat, pumpkin seeds.

Food products or nutritional ingredients whose regular consumption increases the risk of cancer

CANCER TYPE	FOOD PRODUCTS OR FOOD INGREDIENTS
Colorectal cancer	Red meat (beef, pork, mutton) and processed (subjected to smoking, canning, salting or containing added preservatives)
Stomach cancer	Excess salt in the diet
Prostate cancer	Excessive calcium intake with a diet (improperly balanced diet of People practicing sport intensively)
Liver cancer	Foods containing aflatoxins (moldy cereals, nuts, and legumes)
Lung cancer (for smokers)	Beta-carotene used in dietary supplements

Does drinking alcohol cause cancer?

There is a strong link between cancer and alcohol consumption. The strongest connections were found in relation to the upper respiratory tract. Alcohol mainly affects the formation of cancer of the esophagus, throat, and mouth. The mechanisms of alcohol influence on cancer are not fully known, but as alcohol consumption increases, the risk of cancer increases. It is worth limiting alcohol consumption for other health reasons. Frequent drinking causes serious damage to body cells, leading, among others, for cirrhosis, pancreatitis, hypertension, and addiction.

What affects the development of cancer besides diet?

It is important to remember that diet alone is not enough. In addition to it, there are other extremely important factors that affect the risk of cancer. They also include smoking, radiation, environmental pollution, age, low physical activity, viruses and bacteria, tendency to inheritance, occupational factors, some medications.

CHAPTER 5

BREAKFAST RECIPES

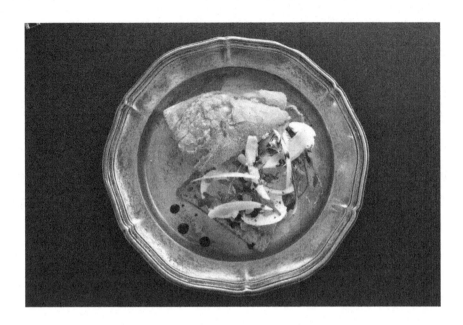

Between dinner and breakfast, being the last and first meals of the day, respectively, there is a long-time interval, which can be from 7 to 10h in some cases. This makes breakfast the most important meal of our day, and regardless of your diet, you should not skip breakfast. He will give us the energy to start our day, as well as provide nutrients and carbohydrates. During our rest, our body burns glucose and glycogen, and it is this reaction that generates energy and maintains the functions of our body, such as circulation, breathing, and heartbeat during sleep, so upon waking, these substances are low and must be replaced. Doing this starts the day with more willingness and greater performance in daily activities. Skipping this meal instead of assisting in weight loss can have the opposite effect since as no food has been eaten, hunger ends up accumulated, and when eating a meal, one tends to eat more than necessary, ingesting greater amount of food and consequently fattening.

Having and maintaining a healthy and balanced diet helps in weight management and provides numerous benefits to our health. The Mediterranean diet is one of the diets with the highest recommendation by nutritionists and specialists. Based on this diet, I created some breakfast options.

For more busy days we have the options:

1. WHOLE TOASTER WITH DAMASK AND YOGHURT

INGREDIENTS

2 tbsp yogurt 1 tbsp honey

3 dried apricots

1 slice whole-wheat toast

PREPARATION METHOD

Cut the apricots in half, place on the slice of whole toast, put the yogurt on the apricots and sweeten with the honey spoon, then serve.

Yield: 1 serving / Degree of difficulty: Easy / Preparation time: 2min To complement this meal, consume 1 fresh seasonal fruit and drink a cup of tea (preferably for herbal infused teas) and can replace the tea with a cup of pure black coffee or latte.

2. MEDITERRANEAN BREAKFAST

INGREDIENTS

1 slice of wholemeal bread

1 slice of minas cheese

1 slice of tomato

Fine herbs to taste

Olive oil thread

Pinch of salt

PREPARATION METHOD

In the slice of brown bread, place the slice of minas cheese and the tomato slice, drizzle with the olive oil, add the herbs according to your taste, and the pinch of salt.

Yield: 1 serving / Degree of difficulty: Easy / Preparation time: 5min As a complement to this meal, eat ½ papaya and drink 1 glass of natural lemon juice, preferably sweetened with demerara sugar or brown sugar.

3. MEDITERRANEAN BREAKFAST (Alternative 2)

INGREDIENTS

1 can of plain nonfat yogurt

2 slices of wholemeal bread

1 medium slice (30g) goat cheese basil or thyme

1 apple or pear

1 glass of natural orange juice

PREPARATION METHOD

Add the whole bread slices with the goat cheese, basil, if you wish to drizzle with a drizzle of olive oil.

Yield: 1 serving / Degree of difficulty: Easy / Preparation time: 5min

4. OMELET WITH SPINACH AND WHITE CHEESE

INGREDIENTS

1 whole egg

3 egg whites

3 tbsp chopped green smelling 1 tsp salt

3 tablespoons butter

1 packet cooked and chopped spinach

200g coarse grated white cheese

8 halved cherry tomatoes

PREPARATION METHOD

1- In a bowl, put the egg whites and egg, beat with the aid of a fouet until the mixture is homogeneous. Add one teaspoon of green smell and half a teaspoon of salt, mix gently, and set aside.

2- In a skillet, melt a tablespoon of butter over medium heat, add the beaten egg mixture, cover the skillet and cook over low heat for 5 minutes or until the eggs are cooked. 3- In a medium saucepan, heat the remaining butter over medium heat. Add the cooked spinach, the white cheese, and the cherry tomatoes, sauté until the cheese has melted, and then add the remaining green smell and half a tablespoon of salt. Stir well and remove from heat.

4 - Spread the filling prepared in the previous step over half of the omelet and, with the help of a spatula, fold the other half over the filling, forming a half-moon. Using the spatula, transfer the omelet from the frying pan to a plate. Serve next and bon appetit!

Yield: 2 servings / Degree of difficulty: Easy / Preparation time: 20min

5. OMELET WITH GARLIC FLATBREAD AND BLACK OLIVES

INGREDIENTS

2 tablespoons olive oil

1 cup of chopped leek

8 cherry tomatoes

¼ cup chopped black olives

1 tbsp chopped fresh rosemary

½ cup pure diced cheese

Salt and pepper to taste

4 eggs

PREPARATION METHOD

Heat a tablespoon of olive oil in a nonstick skillet over medium heat and sauté the leeks until it withers. 2- Add the tomatoes, olives, rosemary, cheese, salt, pepper, and mix, set aside.

In the same skillet, heat the remaining olive oil, pour the eggs lightly beaten with salt and pepper, when still soft, spread the filling, and cook for another 1 minute.

4- Release the sides and fold the omelet forming the half-moon, transfer to another plate, serve next. Enjoy your food!

Yield: 2 servings / Difficulty: Easy / Preparation time: 30min

CHAPTER 6

LUNCH RECIPES

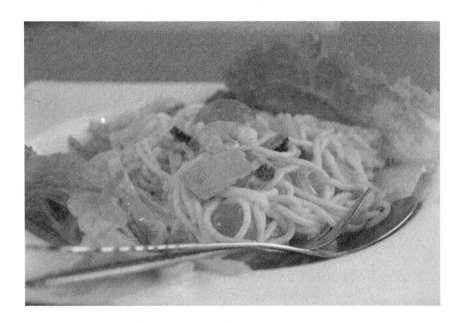

Lunchtime is one of the most important of our day. It is at this meal that we get the most nutrients and calories our body needs. In this meal, we eat foods such as proteins such as meat and fish, vegetables rich in vitamins and fiber, carbohydrates such as rice or pasta, great sources of energy. All of these foods make up a meal that will ensure more energy so we can handle it all day.

Below I will list some main course recipes that are easy and very tasty. These recipes can be performed by anyone who has a minimum of cooking experience. They are nutritious and very low in calories. If consumed in moderate portions, help in weight control. They can be combined with side dishes such as natural juice and a dessert fruit.

6. RATATOUILLE

INGREDIENTS

2 eggplant units

1 unit yellow pepper 1 unit red pepper 2 units zucchini

1 teaspoon salt, full

½ unit diced onion 2 cloves minced garlic

4 pieces of peeled, seedless tomatoes 3 tablespoons chopped parsley

¼ cup extra virgin olive oil

PREPARATION METHOD

1- Cut the eggplant and zucchini into slices of approximately 0.5cm. Reserve.

2- Cut the red and yellow peppers into slices. Reserve.

3. Put eggplant and zucchini slices in a bowl and sprinkle 1 tsp of salt over it. Spread well and let stand for 30min.

4- Drain all the water that forms and dry each eggplant and zucchini slices with a paper towel. Reserve.

5- Heat a skillet well and grease with olive oil.

6 Only grill zucchinis and eggplants. Put a few slices at a time in the pan, being careful not to make them too soft. Reserve them in a container.

In the same skillet, quickly sauté the garlic and onion slices and add the chopped tomatoes. Cook over low heat until tomato begins to crumble.

8- In an ovenproof dish or pan, cover the bottom.

With the braised tomatoes, sprinkle 1 tablespoon chopped parsley and drizzle with about 3 tablespoons extra virgin olive oil.

9- Arrange the slices of vegetables on the platter, interspersing the slices of zucchini, peppers, onion, and eggplant (preferably arrange the vegetables vertically). Drizzle some olive oil over the vegetables.

10— At serving time, bake in preheated oven at 220 ° C for 10min.

Yield: 6 servings / Difficulty: Easy / Preparation time: 80 min

7. ROASTED COD WITH PUNCHED POTATOES

INGREDIENTS

4 cod slices 2 tomatoes

1 yellow pepper

1 red bell pepper

1 green pepper

12 medium potatoes

1 onion

100g pitted black olives

FOR SAUCE - INGREDIENTS

100ml of extra virgin olive oil 50ml of vinegar

Peeled and chopped garlic cloves Salt and ground black pepper to taste

PREPARATION METHOD

1. Desalcate the cod in cold water, changing the water several times.

2. Dry them with a clean cloth.

3. Open the peppers in half and clean them by removing the seeds.

4. Cut the tomatoes into quarters and clean them by removing the seeds.

5. Grill the tomatoes and peppers. Bake the desalted cod slices on the grill.

6. Peel the onion and cut into thin slices. Pass them through flour and remove the excess.

7. Fry them in hot olive oil. Drain them on absorbent paper, removing any excess fat.

8. Bake the peeled potatoes. Once baked, give them a small punch. Potatoes should be cooked but not too soft.

9. Put the indicated sauce ingredients into a glass jar with a lid. Shake it vigorously so that the ingredients mix together.

10. Add the chopped olives.

11. On a platter, place the cod steaks, potatoes, and other ingredients, drizzle with some of the sauce prepared in the previous step, serve very hot!

Tips & Warnings Other vegetables like broccoli can be added to the end of the recipe as long as cooked to the teeth to make the most of their nutrients, steam them.

Yield: 4 servings / Difficulty: Medium / Preparation time: 50 min

8. FETTUCCINE WITH SEA FRUITS AND HERB OLIVE OIL

INGREDIENTS

250g fettuccine 250g squid

6 units of scallop

6 units of clean pink prawns 60g vingo you

100g cherry tomatoes 100g mini zucchini olive oil 200ml Rosemary to taste

1 pack of thyme

1 packet of basil 30g of butter

PREPARATION METHOD

1. Add all the herbs and chop very well with the knife. Add the 150ml olive oil and set aside. The longer it is infused, the better.

2. Clean squids, discarding fins and skin, store bodies, and heads.

3. Fill a large pan with water and bake until boiling, add fettuccine and cook until it is al dente (not too hard and not too soft), at the same time take a large skillet and heat well.

4. Season the shrimps with salt and black pepper, add some of the olive oil to the skillet and place the shrimps, just brown them, without cooking them thoroughly, remove and set aside.

5. Cut the squid body into thin rings, about 0.5cm wide, add the heads and season with salt and black pepper.

6. In the same skillet that the shrimps were sealed, add the clams. They will start cooking, opening, and dropping some water. At this point, add the other seafood, the half-cut cherry tomatoes, and the mini zucchinis. Let it cook for some minutes. Remove from heat.

7. Add the batter with some of the cooking water, and finish with the butter and herbal oil. Mix with seafood and serve immediately.

Yield: 2 servings / Degree of difficulty: Medium / Preparation time: 60 min

9. MEDITERRANEAN OVEN RICE

INGREDIENTS

2 cans of sardines with coconut palm soybean oil (125g each) 2 cups cooked rice

2 small diced seedless tomatoes 1 raw and grated zucchini

100g small diced mozzarella cheese Salt and black pepper to taste

Washed and chopped parsley leaves 5 branches

PREPARATION METHOD

1. In a refractory, add the sardines cut into pieces.

2. Add boiled rice, tomato cubes, grated zucchini, and mozzarella. Season with salt and pepper, mix all ingredients with a fork.

3. Sprinkle some cheese over the whole mixture.

4. Cover with aluminum foil and bake in a medium oven (180 ° C) for approximately 15min, just to warm up.

5. Remove from the oven sprinkle the chopped parsley and then serve.

Yield: 4 servings / Degree of difficulty: Easy / Preparation time: 20min

10. MEDITERRANEAN BOILER

INGREDIENTS

300g pink shrimp 300g squid in rings 300g sea bass

5 units of tomato

2 cloves garlic minced 50ml extra virgin olive oil 30g chopped parsley 50ml dry white wine 100ml fish stock

Salt and black pepper to taste

PREPARATION METHOD

1. In a deep pan, heat extra virgin olive oil, sauté onion and garlic over low heat, let brown.

2. Add tomatoes, white wine and fish stock, season with salt, and cook for about 10 minutes.

3. Add fish first, cook for 3 minutes, then add shrimp and squid, cook for another 3 minutes, or until cooked.

4. Turn off the heat, add the black pepper, the parsley and serve.

Yield: 2 servings / Degree of difficulty: Easy / Preparation time: 25min

CHAPTER 7

ASSORTED SNACKS RECIPES

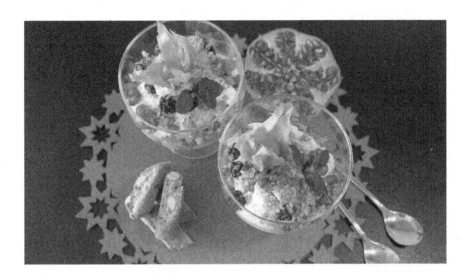

Between lunch and dinner, we have a short time when we don't eat anything, and this is where most people end up sinning because if we don't eat any food in that time, we tend to eat a larger portion during dinner. Therefore, the idea is to keep our body feeling full and, therefore, always having healthy snacks on hand will help us with this task. One tip is always to have a cereal or fruit bar available.

Here are a few snack recipes to follow, which you can make in advance to keep on hand when you need them. They can be carried in a backpack, purse, or lunch box. Besides, many delicious are super nutritious.

11. CEREAL AND DRIED FRUIT BAR

<u>INGREDIENTS</u>

½ cup flaked oats 1 cup granola

½ cup grated coconut

½ cup pistachios (can be substituted for almonds,

peanuts, Brazil nuts, walnuts)

¼ cup flaxseed

2 tablespoons sunflower seeds

¼ cup diced apricots

¼ cup raisins

2 tbsp peanut butter

3 tablespoons honey

1 tablespoon brown sugar

1 teaspoon vanilla

1 pinch of cinnamon

<u>PREPARATION METHOD</u>

1. Preheat oven to 180 ° C, pour dry ingredients mixture into a bowl and mix well. Reserve.

2. Put butter, honey, brown sugar, and vanilla in a small saucepan and bring to a boil. Boil for 30 seconds. Pour the honey mixture over the dry ingredient mixture and stir until uniform.

3. Grease a square baking pan with kitchen spray or line with parchment paper. Pour mixture into baking pan by pressing firmly into baking pan.

4. Bake and bake for 25min. Remove from oven and let cool, carefully slice into bars and refrigerate for at least 2 hours.

5. After this period, individually wrap each bar and store in a refrigerator. Your super healthy and nutritious afternoon snack is ready.

Tips: As an option, you can add or replace with: cardamom, sesame, nutmeg, chocolate powder, dried strawberry, raisin banana, lemon zest, orange zest, walnuts, almonds, etc. You can create your own bar according to your taste. This guarantees a variety of new flavors, always renewing your snack and creating flavors.

Yield: 8 servings / Degree of difficulty: Easy / Preparation time: 180min

12. FULL MUFFINS (STRAWBERRY, BANANA OR APPLE)

INGREDIENTS

Pasta

2 mashed bananas

1 and ½ cup of whole flour

½ cup 1 egg olive oil

Cinnamon to taste

1 tablespoon yeast 3 tablespoons granola

Roof

1 Diced Banana Cinnamon to taste

Peanut butter

Honey, enough to sweeten

PREPARATION METHOD

1. To prepare the dough, mix all the ingredients in an ovenproof dish and place in baking pans. Bake at about 180 ° C for 15min or until a toothpick comes out clean.

2. To make the topping, mix the diced bananas with the peanut butter, honey, and a pinch of cinnamon. If you prefer to use

strawberries or apples instead of bananas, cook them in the microwave oven for 5min or until they soften slightly, then add to the other ingredients.

3. Allow muffins to cool slightly, add topping and serve then.

Tip: You can add or replace it with: almonds, walnuts, chocolates, chia, flaxseed. If you wish, you can fill the muffins with the same mixture used in the topping.

Yield: 6 servings / Degree of difficulty: Easy / Preparation time: 30min

13. OATMEAL COOKIES

INGREDIENTS

175g of flour

½ teaspoon baking powder 85g oatmeal

175g sugar (can be replaced by stevia or brown sugar) 1 tsp cinnamon powder

140g of butter

70g dried blueberries (or raisins) 50g walnuts

1 beaten egg

PREPARATION METHOD

1. Combine flour, baking powder, oats, sugar, and cinnamon in a bowl, mix well with your hands.

2. Add the butter and mix a little more, put the blueberries and walnuts, add the egg and mix well.

3. Lightly sprinkle the table with flour and roll the dough into a cylinder. Wrap in cling film and set aside in the refrigerator until it hardens.

4. Preheat the oven to 160 ° C.

5. Unwrap the dough, cut into thick slices, and place in a baking dish. Bake for 15 minutes or until golden, leave in baking pan until hard.

6. Once cool and hard, store them in a sealed container and just enjoy this super tasty snack.

Yield: 6 servings / Difficulty: Easy / Preparation time: 25min

14. ENERGY GOJI BERRY DATE TRUFFLES

INGREDIENTS

1 cup of pitted dates 3 tablespoons of today's berries

2 teaspoons raw cocoa

2 teaspoons ground cinnamon

½ cup tea of hazelnuts

1 tablespoon chia seeds

<u>PREPARATION METHOD</u>

1. Grind all ingredients in a processor until a compound paste is obtained.

2. Pour the mixture into an ovenproof dish and refrigerate for 30 minutes to 1 hour.

3. Then, using your hands, make small balls the size of truffles or brigadeiros and arrange on a tray.

4. In a saucer, place the cinnamon or raw cocoa and pass the surface of the energy balls to make a layer.

5. Take the refrigerator back and serve whenever you want.

Yield: 10 servings / Degree of difficulty: Easy / Preparation time: 70min

15. FRUIT AND CHEESE SKEWER

<u>INGREDIENTS</u>

Various fruits: kiwi, apple, banana, strawberry, grape, blackberry, blueberry, pineapple, mango, etc.

Cheese

Wooden skewers

PREPARATION METHOD

1. To make this skewer, you will need to cut the fruits into medium cubes or shapes of your choice and stick the skewers, interspersing the fruits with the cheese, keep in the fridge and serve whenever you want.

Tip: This fruit skewer is a great snack to take to work or on a trip for example, as well as being a hit with the kids, you can enjoy the fruits of the seasons and mix with your favorite fruits.

Yield: 6 servings / Difficulty: Very Easy / Preparation Time: 5min

A balanced diet involves not only using high-quality and healthy products for cooking but also following the rules for compiling a daily menu. An integral part of it is the snack. They excite the appetite, so they are usually served at the table before the main dishes. Snacks can be prepared from almost any available product, without spending a lot of time.

The choice of snacks included in the daily or holiday menu depends on which dishes will be served on the first and second. If the main dishes are prepared from fish and meat, then it is advisable to make snacks from vegetables, mushrooms, eggs, cheese, and various pickles. In addition, snacks should be combined with the offered drinks.

Snacks are not only of secondary importance. Many of them are high in calories and may well replace second courses.

16. COLD APPETIZERS OF MEAT PRODUCTS AND POULTRY MEAT APPETIZER WITH MUSHROOMS AND VEGETABLES

INGREDIENTS

Boiled beef - 200g, smoked chicken fillet - 100 g, oyster mushrooms - 100g, mayonnaise - 100g, boiled eggs - 3pcs., Sweet pepper - 1 pcs., Canned green peas - 3 tbsp.s, vegetable oil - 2 tbsp.s, onions - 1 pc., boiled carrots - 1pc., parsley, and cilantro - 0.5 bunches, caraway seeds, salt, ground red pepper to taste.

PREPARATION METHOD

Peel the carrots and cut into circles. The eggs are peeled and chopped. Boiled oyster mushrooms are chopped. Onions and peppers are peeled, cut into rings, mixed with mushrooms, salted, spread in a pan, add oil and fry over medium heat for 10 minutes, then pour in a little water and stew until cooked. Beef and chicken are cut into small slices, salt, pepper, caraway seeds, carrots, eggs, stewed vegetables, and mushrooms are added. All is mixed, seasoned with mayonnaise, laid on a dish in a slide, sprinkled with chopped parsley, decorated with green peas, cilantro sprigs, and served.

17. PUFF APPETIZER WITH LAMB AND FETA CHEESE

INGREDIENTS

Boiled lamb - 300 g, feta cheese - 100 g, boiled rice - 100 g, mayonnaise - 100 g, radish - 5 pcs., Apples - 2 pcs., Parsley root - 1 pc., Raisins - 3 tbsp.s, chopped green cilantro - 1 tbsp, salt.

PREPARATION METHOD

Apples and radishes are peeled and diced, lamb is sliced, and the cheese is rubbed on a coarse grater. Pieces of meat, grated feta cheese, rice, apples, radish, raisins soaked in boiling water and chopped parsley root are laid out in layers on a serving dish. Each layer is salted, greased with mayonnaise. The appetizer is decorated with cilantro and served to the table.

18. CURED MEAT APPETIZER WITH CARROTS

INGREDIENTS

Sun-dried mutton - 300 g, vegetable oil - 70 g, garlic - 2 slices, carrots - 5 pcs., Table vinegar - 2 tbsp.s, adjika - 1 tbsp., caraway seeds, salt, pepper to taste.

PREPARATION METHOD

The peeled carrots are boiled in salted water, knead with a fork, add pre-cooked until soft and sliced dried mutton, salt, adjika diluted in vinegar, crushed garlic, pepper and ground cumin. The appetizer is laid out on a dish and watered with oil.

19. PUFF PASTRY WITH LIVER

INGREDIENTS

Chicken liver - 150 g, canned corn - 2 tbsp.s, mayonnaise - 100 g, butter - 2 tbsp.s, boiled potatoes - 2 pcs., egg - 1 pcs., onions - 2 pcs., tomato - 1 pc., cucumber - 1 pc., chopped celery greens - 3 tbsp.s, breadcrumbs - 1 tbsp., salt to taste.

PREPARATION METHOD

The liver is washed, passed through a meat grinder, fried in 1 tbsp. of oil. Mashed potatoes are made from potatoes with the addition of the remaining oil, salt and beaten egg white. In greased Butter and sprinkled with breadcrumbs spread half the chilled mashed potatoes, then - a layer of fried liver, on top - the remaining mashed potatoes.

Smooth the surface, grease with egg yolk, bake in the oven until golden brown, cool, cut into small pieces and spread on a dish. Sprinkle with chopped onion and pour over mayonnaise. Cucumber and tomato, sliced in circles, are layered on top, greasing each with mayonnaise. The last layer is spread corn and green celery.

20.   MEATLOAF WITH NUTS

INGREDIENTS

Beef - 200 g, chicken fillet - 100 g, chopped walnuts - 2 tbsp.s butter - 2 tbsp.s, vegetable oil - 1 tbsp., salt, pepper.

PREPARATION METHOD

Beef is well beaten, salted, and pepper. Chicken meat is finely chopped. Slices of chicken and a mixture of chopped nuts and vegetable oil are spread on the beef. The meat is rolled, pulled with twine and fried in melted Butter, then cooled and served to the table, cut across the pieces.

21. APPLES STUFFED WITH CHICKEN MEAT AND CHEESE

INGREDIENTS

Apples - 4 pcs., Minced chicken - 200 g, grated cheese - 100 g, butter - 2 tbsp.s, olive oil - 1 teaspoon, salt and pepper to taste.

PREPARATION METHOD

The upper part of apples is cut off, and the core is removed with a special notch. Minced chicken is mixed with Butter, cheese, pepper, and salt. The apples are stuffed with minced meat, placed in a form oiled with olive oil, and baked in a moderately preheated oven for 7-10 minutes.

22. MEAT APPETIZER WITH PEARS

INGREDIENTS

Lamb - 300 g, mayonnaise - 100 g, tomatoes - 3 pcs., Sweet pepper - 2 pcs., Bitter pepper - 1 pod, pears - 2 pcs., Apple - 1 pc., Vegetable oil - 3 tbsp.s, onions - 1 pc., canned green peas - 2 tbsp.s, chopped green onion - 3 tbsp.s, sugar - 1 teaspoon, mustard - 1 teaspoon, parsley - 1 bunch, salt, ground red pepper to taste.

PREPARATION METHOD

Onions and peppers are peeled, cut into rings, washed tomatoes - into slices. The meat is cut into pieces, sprinkled with red ground pepper, fried in oil, mixed with sweet pepper, tomatoes, green peas, and onions.

To prepare the sauce, peeled pears and apples peeled from the skin and core are put in a colander, kept for 5 minutes over a pot of boiling water, then chopped, sugar, mustard, mayonnaise, red pepper, salt, and pieces of hot pepper are added and mixed.

The meat and vegetables is seasoned with sauce, cooled and served to the table, garnished with chopped green onions and parsley.

23.   MEAT AND VEGETABLE CAKE

INGREDIENTS

Boiled beef - 400 g, potatoes - 4 pcs., Carrots - 2 pcs., Grated cheese - 100 g, walnuts 100g, canned green peas - 200 g, mayonnaise - 300 g, pomegranate - 1 pc., salt to taste.

PREPARATION METHOD

Boil potatoes and carrots, peel and rub on a coarse grater, cut the meat into cubes. On a flat dish lay layers of potatoes, carrots, meat, cheese, nuts, green peas. Each layer is salted and greased with mayonnaise. Garnish with pomegranate seeds. The cake is placed in a cool place for 2 hours, then served to the table.

24. CUCUMBER AND JERKY APPETIZER

INGREDIENTS

Sun-dried meat - 100 g, meat broth - 100 ml, sour cream - 100 g, canned green peas - 50 g, cucumbers - 4 pcs., lemon - 1 pc., parsley, chopped dill - 3 tbsp.s, vegetable oil - 1 tbsp., flour - 2 tsp, cilantro - 0.5 bunches, caraway seeds, salt, pepper to taste.

PREPARATION METHOD

Wash cucumbers, cut into thin slices, add dill and juice of half a lemon. To prepare the sauce, the flour is fried in oil; the broth is poured, brought to a boil and kept on low heat until thickened. Then add sour cream, salt, pepper, caraway seeds, bring to a boil, and put parsley greens in the sauce. Prepared cucumbers season with sauce, spread in the middle of the dish with a slide, lay the slices of jerky that are previously boiled to softness at the edges. The appetizer is decorated with slices of the second half of lemon, green peas, cilantro sprigs, and served to the table.

25. TURKISH APPETIZER

INGREDIENTS

Boiled beef - 100 g, cucumber - 1 pc., Tomato - 1 pc., Boiled eggs - 2 pc., Butter - 1 tbsp., grated cheese - 1 tbsp., chopped parsley - 1 teaspoon.

PREPARATION METHOD

Beef is cut into 4 pieces. The eggs are peeled, cut along, the yolks are taken out, the proteins are stuffed with grated cheese, and laid out on pieces of meat. The appetizer is decorated with yolks, crushed with Butter, sliced cucumbers and tomatoes, and served to the table, sprinkled with parsley.

26.   LAMB AND BEANS APPETIZER

INGREDIENTS

String beans - 400 g, boiled lamb - 200 g, mayonnaise - 100 g, pickled cucumbers - 2 pcs., Potatoes - 1 pc., Carrots - 1 pc., Beets - 1 pc., Canned green peas - 1 can, salt pepper.

PREPARATION METHOD

The meat is cut into small pieces. Pre-peeled and cooked individually potatoes, carrots, beets, and green beans are cut into cubes, mixed with green peas and pieces of lamb. Ingredients are salted, pepper and refrigerated for 1 hour. Then add chopped pickles to the snack, season with mayonnaise and serve.

27.   CHICKEN APPETIZER WITH VEGETABLES

INGREDIENTS

Chicken fillet - 700 g, canned green peas - 50 g, mayonnaise - 50 g, pickled cucumbers - 3 pcs., Boiled potatoes - 2 pcs., Boiled carrots - 2 pcs., Olive oil - 2 tbsp.s, boiled eggs - 2 pcs., crushed cilantro greens - 3 tbsp.s, salt to taste.

PREPARATION METHOD

The meat is finely chopped, fried in oil, cooled and combined with sliced cucumbers, potatoes and carrots, chopped eggs and cilantro. The appetizer is salted, seasoned with mayonnaise and served to the table, garnished with green peas.

28.   BEEF HEART APPETIZER

INGREDIENTS

Beef heart - 400 g, boiled rice - 100 g, sour cream - 100 g, onions - 2 pcs., garlic - 3 slices, grated cheese - 3 tbsp.s, vegetable oil - 70 g, table vinegar - 2 tbsp.s, salt, pepper to taste.

PREPARATION METHOD

Beef heart is boiled in salted water with the addition of vinegar, then it is cooled, crushed, mixed with shredded and fried onion, rice and cheese. To prepare the sauce, pre-cleaned garlic is grated on a fine grater, sour cream is added, pepper and mixed. Appetizer seasoned with sauce and served at the table.

29.   LAMB APPETIZER WITH HONEY

INGREDIENTS

Boiled lamb - 200 g, cheese - 200 g, pears - 2 pcs., Boiled potatoes - 1 pc., Tomato - 1 pc., Boiled carrots - 1 pc., Apple juice - 3 tbsp.s, honey - 2 tbsp.s, chopped parsley - 2 tbsp.s.

PREPARATION METHOD

Pre-peeled and sliced pears are mixed with grated potatoes, carrots, and cheese. Add meat and slices of tomato, mix and spread on a dish. The appetizer is poured with apple juice mixed with honey, and served, decorated with parsley greens.

30.   BEEF AND POTATO APPETIZER

INGREDIENTS

Boiled beef - 300 g, boiled potatoes - 2 pcs., Onions - 1 pc., Garlic - 3 slices, mayonnaise - 50 g, chopped parsley - 2 tbsp.s, salt, pepper to taste.

PREPARATION METHOD

The onions are peeled, washed, chopped, mixed with diced potatoes, meat, and pre-peeled and crushed garlic. Salt, pepper, mix, season with mayonnaise and serve, decorated with chopped parsley.

31. LIVER PATE WITH PORK

INGREDIENTS

Beef liver - 500 g, pork - 200 g, butter - 200 g, bacon - 100 g, wheat flour - 2 tbsp.s, onions - 2 pcs., carrots - 1 pc., eggs - 2 pcs., chopped greens - 2 tbsp.s, salt, allspice - 8 pcs., black peas - 8 pcs., ground black pepper to taste.

PREPARATION METHOD

The beef liver is washed, cut into slices, rolled in flour and fried. Pork, peeled carrots, and onions are cut into cubes, put in a pan, peppercorns are added, and stewed until pork is soft. Chilled meat with vegetables and the liver are passed twice through a meat grinder, ground with Butter, beaten eggs are introduced, salt and pepper.

All mix thoroughly and put half finely chopped bacon.

The bottom of the paste form is lined with thinly sliced pieces of bacon, put the cooked mass in the middle, cover it with bacon, and put the dish in the oven for 20-30 minutes.

The prepared paste is cooled, before serving, the mold is slightly heated in hot water and knocked over onto a small plate. Decorate the pate with herbs and serve.

32. SMOKED PHEASANT BREAST PATE WITH BEANS

INGREDIENTS

Smoked pheasant breast - 100 g, beans - 200 g, onions - 1 pc., Vegetable oil - 2 teaspoons, salt, pepper to taste.

PREPARATION METHOD

The pheasant's breast is finely chopped or passed through a meat grinder. Boiled beans, grind or pass through a meat grinder. The onions are peeled, finely chopped and fried in vegetable oil until golden brown. All products are combined, mixed and triturated, salt and pepper are added to taste.

33. RUSTIC SMOKED CHICKEN BREAST PATE

<u>INGREDIENTS</u>

Smoked chicken breast - 150 g, rye bread - 50 g, onion - 1 pc., pepper to taste.

<u>PREPARATION METHOD</u>

Finely chop the breast or pass through a meat grinder, after which it is mixed with peeled and finely chopped onions, pepper is added and thoroughly ground with rye bread.

34. BEEF PASTE IN OIL

<u>INGREDIENTS</u>

Beef paste - 400 g, butter - 120 g, meat jelly - 60 g, boiled eggs - 2 pcs.

<u>PREPARATION METHOD</u>

A layer of softened oil with a thickness of 0.5-0.7 cm is spread on cellophane; the meat paste is spread, the resulting mass is wrapped and put in the refrigerator for some time.

The cooled paste is freed from cellophane, cut into slices with a knife previously dipped in hot water, and decorate each piece with a circle of boiled egg. It is poured over with chilled jelly and refrigerated again to thicken the jelly.

35. CHICKEN MEAT PASTE

INGREDIENTS

Boiled chicken meat - 100 g, butter - 50 g, tomato paste - 1 tbsp., chopped parsley - 1 tbsp., salt, pepper to taste.

PREPARATION METHOD

Chicken meat is passed through a meat grinder. Rub the oil, add chopped herbs, tomato paste, salt, and pepper. All ingredients are thoroughly mixed and cooled.

36. BEEF LIVER PASTE (METHOD 1)

INGREDIENTS

Beef liver - 500 g, bacon - 100 g, butter - 100 g, carrots - 1 pc., Parsley root, 1 pc., Onion - 1 pc., Spices, salt, pepper to taste.

PREPARATION METHOD

The liver is washed, cleaned of films and bile ducts, and cut into small pieces. Peeled carrots, parsley root, and onions are cut into thin slices. All are fried in a pan with bacon, and then twice passed through a meat grinder. Spread the mass in a pan, add salt, pepper, and spices to taste and grind with Butter.

37. BEEF LIVER PASTE (METHOD 2)

INGREDIENTS

Beef liver - 500 g, vegetable oil - 150 g, butter - 70 g, carrots - 1 pc., Onion - 1 pc., salt and pepper to taste.

PREPARATION METHOD

The liver is washed, cut into slices and fried in vegetable oil along with pre-peeled and chopped onions and carrots. All pass through a meat grinder. The mass is mixed with Butter, salt, pepper and beat with a fork or a wooden spatula. The finished paste is transferred to a vase and placed for a while in a cool place.

38. VEAL PASTE IN DOUGH

INGREDIENTS

Veal - 400 g, chicken liver paste - 350 g, tongue - 400 g, bacon - 150 g, meat jelly - 50 g, onion - 1 pc., salt to taste.

For the test: Flour - 200 g, sour cream - 100 g, butter - 75 g, eggs - 3 pcs., Sugar - 1 tbsp., salt to taste.

PREPARATION METHOD

The veal is washed, twice passed through a meat grinder along with peeled onions. The resulting minced meat is combined with a liver paste, salted. The tongue is boiled and cut into cubes.

To prepare a fresh pastry dough, the flour is sifted with a knoll, in the middle they make a recess, put sour cream, Butter, 2 eggs, sugar, salt and quickly knead the dough.

Roll out the dough into a layer with a thickness of 0.5 cm and transfer to a mold. On the dough spread the minced meat with a layer of 2 cm, cut into cubes, boiled tongue, bacon, then again a layer of minced meat (and so on to the top of the form). The last layer of minced meat is covered with dough and the edges are plucked. Grease with a beaten egg on top, make 2-3 round holes with a diameter of 1 cm. Bake in an oven preheated to 180 ° C for 2 hours. Ready paste is cooled without removing from the mold. Then, through the holes made in the dough, pour cold meat jelly and wait until it hardens. After that, remove the paste from the mold and cut into portions.

39.   TURKEY PASTE

INGREDIENTS

Boiled turkey fillet - 300 g, mustard - 40 g, butter - 40 g, egg - 1 pc., onion - 1 pc., Chopped parsley and dill - 2 tbsp.s, salt to taste.

PREPARATION METHOD

Turkey fillet, greens and peeled onions are passed through a meat grinder, an egg is added. Mustard is mixed with Butter. All ingredients are combined, salted, mixed thoroughly and refrigerated for 20 minutes.

40.   CHICKEN LIVER PATE

INGREDIENTS

Chicken liver - 250 g, butter - 150 g, vegetable oil - 50 g, carrots - 1 pc., Onions - 1 pc., Salt, pepper to taste.

PREPARATION METHOD

The peeled carrots and onions, the liver are crushed, fried in vegetable oil, cooled and passed through a meat grinder. Salt, pepper, softened Butter are added to the mass and mixed. Ready paste is put in the refrigerator for 30 minutes.

41. FISH AND SEAFOOD APPETIZERS PICKLED MUSSEL APPETIZER

INGREDIENTS

Mussels - 1 kg, vegetable oil - 50 g, white wine - 100 ml, carrots - 20 g, onions - 1 pc., Lemons - 2 pcs., Celery - 30 g, bay leaf - 1 pc., Chopped dill. - 2 tbsp.s.

PREPARATION METHOD

Mussel shells are cleaned of growths and washed thoroughly. Carrots, celery, onions are peeled, cut into slices, spread in a pan. Mussels are also dropped there. Pour wine, allow on low heat

within 15 minutes before opening the shells. The pan is removed from the stove, the mussels are taken out with a slotted spoon, and both shells are carefully removed.

The broth in which the mussels were cooked is filtered through cheesecloth, the juice squeezed from the lemons, bay leaves are added, and the peeled mussels are poured with this broth.

The pot is put on fire again, cooked broth for 10 minutes with a slight boil. When serving, the mussels are taken out with the vegetables, laid out on a dish, poured with vegetable oil, and sprinkled with herbs.

42.   PICKLED TROUT FILLET

INGREDIENTS

Dried trout - 500 g, carrots - 50 g, onions - 2 pcs., Vegetable oil - 50 g, table wine - 50 ml, mayonnaise - 100 g, table vinegar - 1 tbsp., green salad - 2 sheets, bay leaf - 1 pc., herbs, salt, pepper to taste.

PREPARATION METHOD

Wine, oil, and vinegar are mixed. Cut carrots in circles, onions - in rings, add bay leaf, salt, pepper, wine vinegar mixture, put everything on a stove and bring to a boil. Fish is cut into fillets, poured with hot marinade, and left for 50 minutes. Pickled fillet is taken out with a slotted spoon, spread on a flat dish, circles of carrots and onion rings are spread around, sprinkled with chopped greens, watered with mayonnaise and decorated with lettuce.

CHAPTER 8

DINNER RECIPES

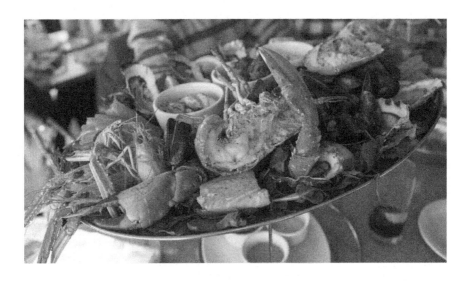

Dinner, in general, should be a lighter meal than lunch; however, it is super important to replenish the energies we spend during our day. Your digestion is often hampered by sleep, so lighter foods such as soups and salads are more recommended than a portion of pasta, for example.

This meal should be taken at least 3 hours before going to bed. It is at dinner that we can insert the wine as an accompaniment. A suggestion is to eat a salmon steak seasoned with lemon, olive oil, and salt, accompanied by grilled vegetables, and a glass of red wine, preferably for dry red wines, because it contains fewer sugars. Another suggestion for dinner is vegetable soup. Herbal tea, such as fennel and chamomile, is indicated before going to bed.

43. GAZPACHO

INGREDIENTS

4 units of red peppers 2 units of green peppers

1 unit of Japanese cucumber 4 units of Debora tomato

½ unit 60ml onion vinegar 30ml lemon juice 90ml olive oil

Salt and black pepper to taste

PREPARATION METHOD

1. Cut off the handle part of the red peppers, open them in half and remove all the seeds, also removing the white part where the seeds are. Cut the peppers into smaller pieces, set aside.

2. Remove the peel from the cucumber. Cut in half and remove seeds, cut each half into 3 pieces, and set aside.

3. Take the tomatoes, remove only the center of the tomato and cut into smaller pieces, set aside.

4. Peel the onion peel, cut it into pieces, and set aside.

5. Put all of the above ingredients into the blender, add the lemon juice, vinegar, and olive oil and beat well. When all the ingredients are well ground and mixed, strain to a very fine chinois.

6. Refrigerate to cool. At the serving time, set the salt and pepper seasoning and always serve well chilled.

Yield: 2 servings / Degree of difficulty: Easy / Time to preparation: 20min

44. CARROT, ORANGE, HONEY AND CORIANDER CREAM

INGREDIENTS

Cream

800g sliced carrot 1.5 liters potato cream Salt to taste

50ml olive oil 100ml orange juice

Side dish

300g of orange 25g of coriander 100ml of honey

Olive oil to taste

PREPARATION METHOD

1. In a glass container, place the carrots, season with olive oil, salt, black pepper, and orange juice. Cook in microwave oven for about 10min or until carrots are cooked.

2. Blend in the potato cream blender, check the seasoning and, if necessary, adjust the salt and black pepper. Reserve.

Side dish

1. For garnish, degrease the orange by removing the seeds. Reserve.

2. Separate some coriander leaves and honey.

3. Serve the cream in a deep dish with the orange slices, coriander leaves, and honey.

Yield: 4 servings / Degree of difficulty: Easy / Preparation time: 30min

45.   FULL RICE WITH LENTIL AND BASIL

INGREDIENTS

4 tablespoons butter 2 cloves garlic, crushed

½ cup of rice

½ cup of lentil

½ cup dry white wine

½ teaspoon salt

2 cups boiling water

3 tablespoons chopped fresh basil

PREPARATION METHOD

1. In a pan, heat the 2 tablespoons of butter over medium heat, sauté the garlic, wait until golden brown.

2. Add rice and lentil and sauté for another 3 minutes, constantly stirring so that it does not burn.

3. Add the wine, salt, and cook for another 3 minutes or until the wine has evaporated.

4. Add water and lower the heat. Cover the pan and cook for another 35 minutes or until all the water has dried.

5. Add the basil and the remaining butter and mix gently.

6. Set aside for 5 minutes and serve then.

Yield: 6 servings / Degree of difficulty: Easy / Preparation time: 60min

46. MEDITERRANEAN HOT SALAD

<u>INGREDIENTS</u>

200g swine leg

2 units red onion 1 packet of arugula

2 tomato units

½ cup black tea Olive oil to taste

Balsamic Aceto to taste Parmesan in chips to taste

Marinade

40ml of lemon juice

¼ cup olive oil 1 tsp oregano 1 clove garlic

<u>PREPARATION METHOD</u>

1. To make the marinade, place all ingredients in a capped glass jar and shake vigorously until all ingredients are well mixed, set aside.

2. Cut the ham into thin slices and season with the marinade. Let it sit for a few hours. The longer the ham is enjoying the marinade, the more delicious it gets.

3. Peel the onion and cut it into petals, set aside.

4. Remove the stone from the olives and cut the tomatoes in medium cubes.

5. Remove the ham from the marinade and remove excess moisture with a paper towel.

6. Heat a pan, lightly brown the ham and set aside.

7. In the same pan add a little olive oil and saute the onion, when they are translucent, add the olives, turn the ham and stir for a few moments.

8. In a deep bowl, mix arugula and tomato with ham and onion, season with balsamic, stir well, and add parmesan chips.

9. Serve next.

Yield: 2 servings / Degree of difficulty: Easy / Preparation time: 90min

47.   ARTICHOKE BACKGROUND WITH HERB PASTE

INGREDIENTS

½ teaspoon white pepper 2 tsp salt

½ glass of white wine 3 bay leaves

2 cloves garlic 2 liters of water

4 units artichoke bottom

2 tablespoons chopped basil 2 tablespoons chopped parsley

½ cup fresh cream milk 200g cream cheese

1 tbsp chopped green onions Salt and black pepper to taste

4 tablespoons grated Parmesan

PREPARATION METHOD

1. Using a knife and scissors remove all artichoke leaves and bristles, leaving only the bottom of the artichoke.

2. Then put the water, salt, black pepper, wine, garlic, and bay leaf in a deep pan and leave the bottom of the artichoke cook until tender. Reserve.

Filling

1. Mix the cream cheese with the cream until it forms a paste.

2. Add parsley, basil, chives, salt, and pepper, mix well.

3. Pass this paste over the artichoke.

4. Place the artichoke with the paste in a baking dish and sprinkle the Parmesan on top, granite over medium to high heat for about 10 minutes.

5. Allow to cool for a few minutes and serve then.

Yield: 4 servings / Degree of difficulty: Easy / Preparation time: 60min

CHAPTER 9

DESSERTS RECIPES

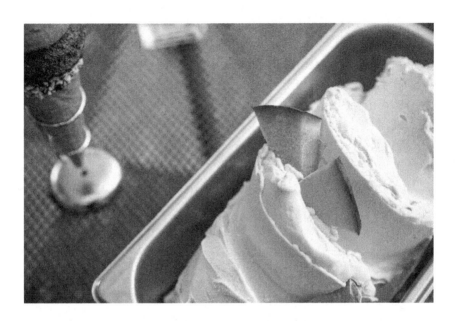

Desserts can be included in the diet provided in moderation and in small portions. Some of the following recipes are based on nonfat yogurt and fruits, as well as cereals, nuts, and walnuts, which ensures a healthy and tasty dessert.

Avoid temptation and consume very high-calorie, high-sugar desserts, such as chocolate and ice cream cakes, avoid industrialized cakes, and always prefer one that has fruits and cereals, such as the walnut and blueberry yogurt parfait available below.

48.   DAMASCO LIGHT DESSERT

INGREDIENTS

100g of ricotta light

100g of light cream 100g of nonfat yogurt 2 tablespoons honey

100g of dried apricots

PREPARATION METHOD

1. In a blender beat the ricotta, sour cream, yogurt, and honey, until smooth, set aside.

2. Apricots need to be soaked for at least 2 hours to make them soft, so put them in a bowl of enough water to cover them.

3. After 2 hours, beat the apricots with the water in which it was soaked in a blender until it becomes a kind of puree.

4. Place the cream prepared in the first step into cups or bowls, add a spoonful of the puree prepared in the previous step over each cup or bowl, refrigerate and let it harden a little. Your dessert is ready.

Apricots can be replaced by dates or plums. Honey, however, can be replaced by demerara or brown sugar.

Yield: 4 servings / Degree of difficulty: Easy / Preparation time: 2h30min

49. FRUIT YOGHURT

<u>INGREDIENTS</u>

Fruits to taste (apple, banana, strawberry, plum) 100g of nonfat yogurt

2 tablespoons Granola honey to taste

<u>PREPARATION METHOD</u>

1- Chop the fruits of your choice (suggestion: give preference to seasonal fruits, strawberry, plum, banana, and apple, are good options), choose from one or more fruits.

2- In a bowl mix a layer of the chopped fruits and the nonfat yogurt, repeat this procedure until the bowl is complete if you want to sweeten finish with a spoon of honey and granola.

Yield: 2 servings / Difficulty: Easy / Preparation time: 5min

50. SWEET LIGHT RICE

<u>INGREDIENTS</u>

½ cup brown rice 500ml skim milk 1 lemon

Cinnamon sticks

Stevia Sweetener Corn Starch

PREPARATION METHOD

1- Put the rice on the fire with two cups of water, 2 sticks in sticks and 5 cloves, after the water is almost dry, gradually add the skim milk. When you feel boiled rice, feel the thin broth, dissolve one dessert spoon of cornstarch in two spoons of skimmed milk and toss in the rice.

2- Add the stevia sweetener in powder or liquid (can be replaced by demerara sugar) check the taste not over to sweeten, when it reaches the point, throw the zest of a lemon peel, leave for another 3 minutes and turn off the heat.

3- Serve with cinnamon powder on top, hot or cold.

Yield: 4 servings / Degree of difficulty: Easy / Preparation time: 1 hour

51. LIGHT PAPAYA CREAM

INGREDIENTS

½ papaya

1 cup of nonfat yogurt 1 cup with ice and water

PREPARATION METHOD

1. Peel the papaya and put it in a blender

2. Beat the papaya pulp with the other ingredients in a blender, and you're done.

Tip: Serve ice cream with fresh, sweet fruits such as berries, such as blackberry, raspberry, and blueberry. The nonfat yogurt can be replaced by 3 tablespoons of cream or sour cream.

Yield: 2 servings / Difficulty: Easy / Preparation time: 5min

52. YOGURT PARFAIT WITH BLUE AND WALNUT PECAN

INGREDIENTS

1 cup cold cooked quinoa

2 cups of Greek yogurt (original recipe uses vanilla-flavored yogurt)

2 cups blueberry

¼ cup pecan nuts 1 tbsp honey

PREPARATION METHOD

1. Cook one cup of quinoa in two cups of water, cooking it until water is absorbed. Let cool.

2. In a bowl, overlap the quinoa layers, followed by one of yogurt, blueberry, and walnuts until the bowl is fully filled.

3. Sprinkle the top with the honey. Enjoy your food! Tip: serve ice cream if you prefer.

Yield: 4 servings / Degree of difficulty: Easy / Preparation time: 15min

CHAPTER 10

MEDITARRANEAN PIZZA RECIPES

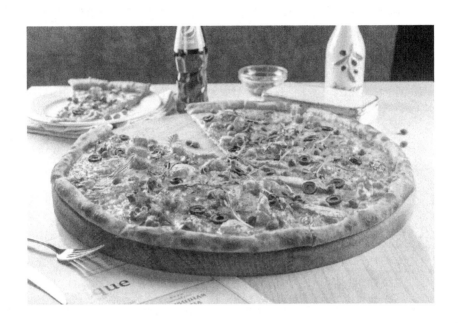

53. PIZZA WITH LAMB AND TOMATOES

<u>INGREDIENTS</u>

For the test: 200 g flour, 20 g sugar, 135 g butter, 1 egg.

For the filling: 250 g of rice, 1 onion, 250 g of lean lamb, 200 g of cheese, 1 egg, 3 cloves of garlic, 5 tomatoes, ground black pepper, salt to taste.

PREPARATION METHOD

Knead the puff pastry, place for half an hour in the cold. Then roll out and put on a baking sheet. Pre-boil rice cut the lamb into strips, and the onion into rings. Finely chop the garlic and egg. Mix all the ingredients, salt, and pepper to taste, put on the dough: peel and mash tomatoes. Cover the filling with the resulting tomato paste. Grate the cheese on a grater — Bake in a hot oven for 30 minutes.

54.   PIZZA WITH BOILED BEEF

INGREDIENTS

For the test: 250 grams of flour, 25 grams of yeast, 50 grams of butter, 2 teaspoons of sugar, 2 eggs, 0.5 cups of milk, 0.5 teaspoons of salt.

For the filling: 500g lean boiled beef, 4 pickled cucumbers, 1 pod of sweet pepper, 1 hard-boiled egg, 0.5 tbsp.s of wine vinegar, 4 tbsp.s of mayonnaise.

PREPARATION METHOD

Cook the yeast dough, roll out and put on a greased baking sheet. Slice the beef into strips and place on the dough. Cut the cucumbers into strips, pepper - in half rings, tomatoes - in slices. Chop onion finely. Mix vegetables and season with vinegar. Put the vegetable mixture on the meat. Grease with mayonnaise. Garnish with egg slices on top. Bake in a hot oven for 20 minutes.

55. PIZZA WITH BOILED LOIN

<u>INGREDIENTS</u>

For the test: 250g flour, 25g yeast, 1 cup milk, 2 eggs, 1 tbsp. of sugar, 0.5 teaspoon of salt, 3 tbsp.s of vegetable oil.

For the filling: 200 g of boiled loin and brown sauce.

For sauce: 2 tbsp.s of fat, 2 tbsp.s of flour, 0.5 l of broth, 1–2 tsp of butter (1-2 tbsp of cream or sour cream), fruit puree, pepper and salt to taste.

<u>PREPARATION METHOD</u>

To prepare the sauce, warm the fat, brown the flour in it. As a liquid, a cubed broth can be used. Cook for 6-8 minutes. Then season with butter, add sour cream or cream if desired. Add fruit puree to the sauce a few minutes before the end of cooking. Sauce season with sugar. Allow to cool.

Cook the yeast dough, let it come, knead it again and put on a greased baking sheet. Cut the loin into thin strips or slices, put in a dish and pour half the sauce. Allow to stand for 5 minutes, put on the prepared dough and pour the remaining sauce.

56.   PIZZA WITH ITALIAN GLAZE

INGREDIENTS

250 g flour, 25 g yeast, 1 cup milk, 2 eggs, 1 tbsp. of sugar, 0.5 teaspoon of salt, 3 tbsp.s of vegetable oil.

For the filling: 300 g of smoked meat (carbonate, bacon, loin, neck, smoked chicken), prunes, olive oil, Italian glaze.

PREPARATION METHOD

Finely chop the garlic and onion to make the glaze. Blanch the tomatoes, peel and finely chop. Put oil and tomatoes on low heat. Sugar diluted in 1 tbsp. of water and mix with tomato Add the chopped mixture of garlic and onions and warm again. Add curry powder to the mixture. Cool and let it brew.

Prepare the yeast dough, let it come, knead it again and put it on a baking sheet, greased with olive oil. Sprinkle the dough again with butter. Finely chop the smoked meats, lay them on the cooked test. Sprinkle the prunes with boiling water, chop and lay on top of the smoked meats. Put in the oven for 30 minutes. Reach, add glaze and bake for another 10 minutes.

57. PIZZA CAKE

<u>INGREDIENTS</u>

2 cups flour, 0.7 cups milk, 0.35 cups vegetable oil, 1 tbsp. of baking powder or 1 teaspoon (without top) of baking soda, extinguished with vinegar.

For the filling: 500 g of hard grated cheese, 1 large or 2 medium onions, a little caviar oil, 200 g of tomato paste, 150-200 g of non-fat smoked meats, 2-3 hard-boiled eggs, 150-200 g of mushrooms, 1 tbsp. of butter or creamy margarine, a pinch of camphor basil. For decoration: parsley, 1 tomato, sprats, etc.

<u>PREPARATION METHOD</u>

Thoroughly combine milk, vegetable oil (beat with a mixer), add flour, baking powder, salt. Knead the dough (it should be the same consistency as the shortbread). Grease a large baking dish with vegetable oil, cover its bottom and sides with dough. Spread the fillings evenly in the following order:

layer - the fourth part of grated hard cheese; layer - onion, sliced in thin circles; layer - caviar oil (if any);

layer - pour camphor basil; layer - half a portion of tomato paste; layer - thin slices of smoked meats;

layer - a quarter of the norm of grated hard cheese;

layer - hard-boiled eggs, sliced in circles, slightly salted and sprinkled with pepper;

layer - champignons (previously stewed in 1 tbsp. of butter);

layer - the remaining tomato paste; layer - the remaining hard cheese;

layer - external design: pieces of tomato, small pieces of canned fish in tomato sauce, small mushrooms soaked in vegetable oil and sprigs of parsley.

Cover (e.g., with aluminum foil) and bake in a well-heated oven for 30 minutes. Such pizza can be prepared in advance (for example, before guests arrive), keeping a few teas in the refrigerator, and then baking before serving.

58.   PIZZA WITH BACON AND CAULIFLOWER

INGREDIENTS

For the test: 250 g flour, 0.5 cups sour cream, 2 teaspoons of sugar, 2 eggs, 50 g of butter, 0.5 teaspoon of salt.

For the filling: 200 g of bacon, 600 g of low-fat cottage cheese, 300 g of cauliflower, 2 eggs, 2 carrots, 1 onion, pepper and salt to taste.

PREPARATION METHOD

Cook the puff pastry, roll out and put in a baking dish greased with fat. Dice the bacon and put on the dough. Cut carrots and onions into circles, mix and add cauliflower. Add salt and pepper to taste. Put a layer on the bacon. Mix the cottage cheese with eggs and cover the surface of the pizza with this mixture. Place in a hot oven and bake for 25-30 minutes.

59. ROYAL PIZZA

INGREDIENTS

For the test: 250 g flour, 25 g yeast, 1 cup milk, 2 eggs, 1 tbsp. of sugar, 0.5 teaspoon of salt, 3 tbsp.s of vegetable oil.

For the filling: 500 g of tomatoes, 200 g of boiled ham, 2 tbsp.s of olive oil, 100 g grated cheese, 12 olives, pepper and salt to taste.

PREPARATION METHOD

Cook the yeast dough, let it come, knead it again and put on a greased baking sheet. Peel the tomatoes and cut into slices. Cut ham into thin strips. Lay tomatoes and ham on layers of dough. Top with olives. Sprinkle with pepper and grated cheese. Bake in the oven for 35 minutes.

60.   PIZZA "CAPRICCIOSA"

<u>INGREDIENTS</u>

For the test: 250 g flour, 20 g yeast, 1 cup milk, 2 eggs, 1 tbsp. of sugar, 0.5 teaspoon of salt, 3 tbsp.s of vegetable oil.

For the filling: 300 g of peeled tomatoes, 400 g of ham, sliced in thin slices, 4 thin slices of Swiss cheese, 300 g of champignons, 1 teaspoon of garlic, 1 cup of white wine, 1 tbsp. of vegetable oil, salt to taste.

<u>PREPARATION METHOD</u>

Cook the yeast dough, let it come, knead it again and put on a greased baking sheet. To chopped champignons add 1 tbsp. of vegetable oil, a clove of garlic, a glass of white wine and cook for 15 minutes. To salt. Grease the dough with butter and cover with chopped tomatoes, slices of ham, mushrooms and slices of cheese. Put in a preheated oven and bake for 20 minutes.

61. PIZZA WITH HAM
<u>INGREDIENTS</u>

For the test: 200 g of flour, 10 g of yeast, 0.5 cup of milk, 1 teaspoon of sugar, 0.5 teaspoon of salt, 1 tbsp. of vegetable oil.

For the filling: 2 dill roots, 200 ml of vegetable broth, 6 tbsp.s finely chopped green onions, 300 g fat sour cream. 4 tbsp.s of grated cheese, 5-6 small tomatoes, 200 g of boiled ham, ground black pepper and salt to taste.

PREPARATION METHOD

Knead the yeast dough on a dough, let it come up, knead thoroughly again, roll it into a 5 mm thick layer and put on a greased baking sheet. Roots Rinse dill thoroughly, peel and cut into small slices. Boil in vegetable broth. Mix onion, sour cream and grated cheese. Season with salt and pepper to taste. Lubricate the dough with sour cream, sprinkle with finely chopped ham. Put tomatoes and dill roots on top. Place in a hot oven for 20 minutes.

62.   PIZZA WITH SALAMI

INGREDIENTS

For the test: 250 g flour, 25 g yeast, 1 cup milk, 2 eggs, 1 tbsp. of sugar, 0.5 teaspoon of salt, 3 tbsp.s of vegetable oil.

For the filling: 100 g Swiss cheese, 8 olives, 200 g champignons, 2 tomatoes, 200 g salami with garlic, 200g grated Edamer cheese, 1 tbsp. of butter or margarine, 2 tbsp.s of vegetable oil, oregano and salt to taste.

PREPARATION METHOD

Cook the yeast dough, let it come, knead it again and place on a greased baking tray. Sprinkle the dough with butter. Slice the cheese. Cut the pitted olives in half. Peel and chop mushrooms, fry in a small amount of butter. Dice tomatoes and salami. Cover the dough with cheese, put olives in the middle, arrange the remaining components of the filling around. Sprinkle with salt and oregano, then grated cheese and put in a preheated oven for 15 minutes.

63.   PIZZA "CALZONE"

<u>INGREDIENTS</u>

For the test: 200 g flour, 10 g yeast, 0.5 cup milk, 1 teaspoon sugar, 0.5 teaspoon salt, 1 tbsp. of vegetable oil.

For the filling: 200 g salami, 300 g hard cheese, 100 g soft cheese, 2 tbsp.s of marjoram, 4 eggs, 4 tbsp.s grated Swiss cheese, 5 tbsp.s of olive oil, 4 tbsp.s mashed tomatoes, 1 tbsp. of herbal mixture, ground black pepper and salt to taste.

<u>PREPARATION METHOD</u>

Prepare the yeast dough on a dough in double quantity. Roll 4 identical circles. Grate hard cheese, then mix with marjoram and eggs. Add salt and pepper to taste. Soft cheese and salami cut into cubes, mix with 2 tbsp.s of Swiss cheese and add to the cheese mass. Lubricate the pan and lay out the dough circles. Grease the dough with butter. Divide the filling into 4 parts and lay out each one in one half of the circle. Cover with the other half. Fasten the edges of the dough tightly. Lubricate the pizza with the rest of the butter and lay the mashed tomatoes. Sprinkle with herbs. Place in a hot oven and bake for 20 minutes.

64. TARANTELLA PIZZA

INGREDIENTS

For the test: 250 g flour, 25 g yeast, 1 cup milk, 2 eggs, 1 tbsp. of sugar, 0.5 teaspoon of salt, 3 tbsp.s of vegetable oil.

For the filling: 18 sausages or sausages in juice, 200 g of boiled, finely chopped meat, tomato puree, 100 g of grated Swiss cheese, 3 tbsp.s of olive oil, 100 g olives (to taste).

PREPARATION METHOD

Cook the yeast dough, let it come, knead it again and put on a greased baking sheet. Sprinkle the dough with butter. Put meat on top, spread tomato puree, evenly distribute sausages and olives and sprinkle with cheese. Sprinkle with oil and bake in the oven.

65. PIZZA IN A RUSTIC WAY

INGREDIENTS

For the test: 300 g of potatoes, 300 g of flour, 50 g of butter or margarine, 2 tbsp.s of grated cheese, 1 egg, 20 g of yeast, 0.5 cups of milk, pepper and salt to taste.

For the filling: 50 g of cooked sausage, 50 g of ham, 3 processed cheese, 50 g of cheese, 3 tbsp.s of grated cheese, 2 eggs, 1 cup of milk, pepper and salt to taste.

PREPARATION METHOD

Boil potatoes in a peel, peel it, knead on a table or board, mix thoroughly with flour. Centre make a hole, pour in an egg, dissolved butter or margarine, sprinkle with grated cheese, salt, pepper, pour in yeast diluted with warm milk. Knead the tender dough, cover it with a towel and place in a warm place for 2 hours. Then roll it out and put it on a pan with a diameter of 24-26 cm, 5 cm high, greased with butter, so as to cover the bottom and walls of the pan.

In a bowl put finely chopped sausage, ham, cheese, cheese, grated cheese, pour eggs and milk, salt, pepper and beat well. Put the filling on the dough, close it on the edges, put in the hot oven for 40-50 minutes. Serve hot.

66. PIZZA WITH SAUSAGES AND TOMATOES

INGREDIENTS

For the test: 250g flour, 50g butter or margarine, 25 g yeast, 1 cup milk, 0.5 teaspoon salt.

For the filling: 500 g sausages, 1 onion, 450 g peeled tomatoes, 1 clove of garlic, butter, parsley, black pepper and salt to taste.

PREPARATION METHOD

Stir finely chopped sausages, onions and parsley. Put the mixture in a layer 2 cm thick in a clay bowl, grated with a clove of garlic and greased with butter, and put without a lid in a hot oven for 20-25 minutes.

Sift flour on a table, make a hole, add prepared yeast, salt, mix thoroughly, add small pieces of butter or margarine, warm milk, put in a warm place for 2 hours. Roll out a 2 cm thick circle.

Remove the bowl with the mixture from the oven, put finely chopped tomatoes seasoned with salt and black ground pepper on top, lay a circle of tomatoes on the tomatoes, press the dough along the edges. Lubricate with dissolved butter and put in a very hot oven for 15-20 minutes.

67. PIZZA WITH TURKEY

INGREDIENTS

For the test: 200 g of flour, 10 g of yeast, 0.5 cups of milk, 1 teaspoon of sugar, 0.5 teaspoon of salt, 1 tbsp. of vegetable oil.

For the filling: 600 g mashed tomatoes, 1 tbsp. of marjoram, 1 pod of sweet pepper, 1 can of canned red beans and corn, 150 g of sheep's cheese, 600 g of turkey breast, 1 tbsp. of vegetable oil, 50 g of grated Chester cheese.

PREPARATION METHOD

Knead the yeast dough on a dough, roll into a 5 mm thick layer and put on a baking sheet. Mix grated tomatoes with spices, add a little oil and heat in a pan. Cut bell pepper and mix with beans and corn. Add the diced sheep's cheese. Finely chop the turkey meat and fry in oil, salt. Put tomatoes on the dough, then meat and vegetables. Sprinkle with grated cheese and place in the oven for 20 minutes.

68.   PIZZA "TUSCANY"

INGREDIENTS

For the test: 250 g flour, 150 g butter, 2 eggs, 2 tbsp.s of sugar, salt.

For the filling: 400 g of roasted turkey fillet, 2 grapefruits, 3 carrots, 200 g of zucchini, 1 cup mixed, pepper and salt to taste.

<u>PREPARATION METHOD</u>

Knead the puff pastry, roll out and put on a greased baking sheet. Finely chop the turkey meat and lay it evenly on the dough. Season with spices. Peel the grapefruits, remove the skin and squeeze the juice slightly. Cover the turkey meat with a layer of pulp. Sprinkle grated carrots on top, then zucchini. Pour sour cream into the dish, put in the oven and bake for 20-25 minutes.

69. PIZZA WITH CHICKEN AND MAYONNAISE

<u>INGREDIENTS</u>

For the test: 200g flour, 10 g yeast, 0.5 cup milk, 1 teaspoon sugar, 0.5 teaspoon salt.

For the filling: 1 boiled chicken, 3-4 ripe tomatoes, 6 tbsp.s of mayonnaise, 2-3 cloves of garlic, 1 tsp a chock of sweet pepper, 2 small carrots, 0.5 onions, 50 g butter, dill and parsley to taste.

<u>PREPARATION METHOD</u>

Prepare the yeast dough from the indicated quantity of products and roll into a circle with a diameter of 50 cm. Chop the onion and carrots finely and fry until cooked. Uniformly put on the dough. Separate the chicken pulp from the bones and chop. Put the next layer on the pizza, and then chop the tomatoes and bell peppers coarsely. Mix mayonnaise and chopped garlic and grease pizza with it. Place in a hot oven for 20 minutes. Decorate the finished pizza on top with chopped herbs.

70.   PIZZA WITH CHICKEN AND CHEESE

INGREDIENTS

For the test: 200 g flour, 10 g yeast, 0.5 cup milk, 1 teaspoon sugar, 0.5 teaspoon salt.

For the filling: 1 boiled chicken, 4 hard-boiled eggs, 3 potatoes, 2 carrots, 2-3 unsweetened apples, 100 g of cheese, 2 tbsp.s of olive oil.

PREPARATION METHOD

Prepare the yeast dough in the indicated proportion and place on a greased baking sheet. Chicken, cut into 3 equal portions. Peel potatoes and carrots and cut into slices 3-5 mm thick. Peel the apples, remove the core, chop finely. Put a third of the chicken in a thin layer on the dough, lay the chopped eggs on top, then potatoes and carrots, again a portion of chicken, apples, the last portion of chicken. Sprinkle everything with grated cheese, pour olive oil. Place the baking tray with pizza in a hot oven and bake for 25-30 minutes.

71. PIZZA WITH CHICKEN LIVER

INGREDIENTS

For the test: 200 g flour, 10 g yeast, 0.5 cup milk, 1 teaspoon sugar, 0.5 teaspoon salt, 1 tbsp. of vegetable oil.

For the filling: 300 g chicken liver, 2 tomatoes, 3 tbsp.s of olives, 2 onions, 4 tbsp.s of mayonnaise, pepper and salt to taste.

PREPARATION METHOD

Cook the yeast dough and place on a greased baking sheet. Cut the liver into small pieces, and the onion into rings, mix and add half the olives. Put on the dough. Peel and mash tomatoes, season with salt and pepper to taste. Put the tomato puree on the liver. Lubricate with mayonnaise on top and garnish with the remaining olives. Bake in the oven for 20-25 minutes.

72. PIZZA SICILIAN

INGREDIENTS

For the test: 250 g flour, 25 g yeast, 1 cup milk, 2 eggs, 1 tbsp. of sugar, 0.5 teaspoon of salt, 3 tbsp.s of vegetable oil.

For the filling: 6 anchovies in oil, onions, tomato paste, 3 tomatoes, 100 g of grated Edamer cheese, 50 ml of olive oil, salt to taste.

PREPARATION METHOD

Cook the yeast dough, let it come, knead it again and place on a round baking sheet, oiled. Make indentations in the test, in which to place the anchovies. Grease the top with tomato paste, sprinkle with finely chopped onions, cover with tomato slices, salt, sprinkle with cheese, drizzle with butter and place in the oven for 30 minutes.

73.   PIZZA WITH TUNA AND OLIVES

INGREDIENTS

For the test: 200 g of flour, 10 g of yeast, 0.5 cup of milk, 1 teaspoon of sugar, 0.5 teaspoon of salt, 1 tbsp. of vegetable oil.

For the filling: 4 cloves of garlic, 4 onions, 1 kg of tomatoes, 2 tbsp.s of grated Swiss cheese, 300 g of tuna fish in vegetable oil, 32 olives, 300 g of grated cheese, pepper and salt to taste.

PREPARATION METHOD

Prepare the yeast dough on a dough and put on a greased baking sheet. Peel and finely chop the garlic. Mix thoroughly with slices of tomatoes and Swiss cheese. Add salt and pepper to taste. Place the tuna meat in a sieve, drain and separate.

CHAPTER 11

MEDITERRANEAN SALAD RECIPES

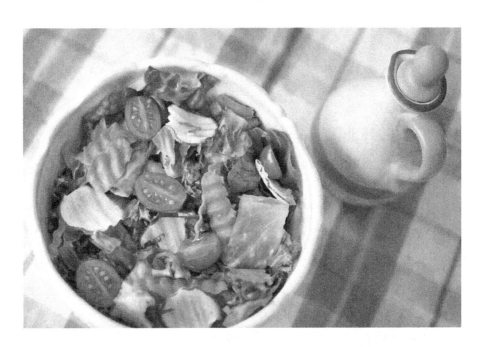

74. CHICKEN SALAD WITH VEGETABLES IN HONEY SAUCE

5 servings

Calorie content 1 serving - 130 kcal Cooking time - 15min

INGREDIENTS

Boiled chicken fillet - 200 g Cheese - 200 g Apples - 200g Tomatoes - 100g

Boiled carrots - 100 g Apple juice - 15 ml Honey - 20g

Shredded parsley - 20g

PREPARATION METHOD

1. Pre-peeled and sliced apple mix with grated carrots and cheese.

2. Add finely chopped chicken meat and sliced tomatoes to the prepared ingredients, salt, mix and put on a dish

3. To prepare the sauce, combine apple juice with honey, curry, and pepper. Lettuce pours the mixture obtained, decorate with parsley, and serve.

75. BEEF AND RADISH SALAD

5 servings

Calorie content 1 serving - 80 kcal Cooking time - 15 min

INGREDIENTS

Boiled beef - 100 g radish - 200g

Onions - 100g

Shredded walnuts - 30 g Low-calorie mayonnaise - 150 g Vegetable oil - 20 ml Dill and parsley - 30g Sha salt to taste

PREPARATION METHOD

1. Cut the meat into small pieces

2. Peel and grate the radish.

3. Chop the onion finely, put the stew in a frying pan and fry eV vegetable oil.

4. Mix all the ingredients, add most of the nuts, salt, pepper, and season with mayonnaise.

5. Before serving, sprinkle lettuce with finely chopped parsley and dill. Garnish with the remaining nuts.

76.   RABBIT MEAT SALAD WITH CELERY

5 servings

Calorie content in 1 portion - 70 kcal Cooking time - 10 min

INGREDIENTS

Roasted rabbit meat - 250 g Celery roots - 100 g Seedless olives - 100 g

Pickled cucumbers - 300 g Eggs - 2 pcs.

Spur red sweet - 1 pc. Lemon juice - 30 ml

Low-calorie mayonnaise - 50 g Butter - 50 g

Sugar - 5 g

Parsley - 5 g Salt and pepper to taste

PREPARATION METHOD

1. Cut rabbit meat into strips.

2. Grind the peeled celery roots and fry in butter until soft

3. Peel and chop the cucumbers.

4. Hard-boiled eggs, peel them, cut into 8 pieces each

5. Combine all ingredients, sprinkle with lemon juice, add sugar, salt, and pepper.

6. Salad season with mayonnaise, garnish with olives, sprigs of parsley and sliced pepper

77. CHICKEN SALAD WITH BOILED VEGETABLES

5 servings

Calorie content 1 serving - 112 kcal Cooking time - 25 min

INGREDIENTS

Chicken fillet - 500 g

Canned green peas - 50 g Low-calorie mayonnaise - 50 g

Pickled cucumbers - 3 pcs. Boiled potatoes - 200 g

Boiled carrots - 200 g Olive oil - 20 ml Boiled eggs - 2 pcs.

Salt to taste

PREPARATION METHOD

1. Finely chop the fillet, fry in oil, cool and combine with sliced cucumbers, cubes of potatoes and carrots and chopped eggs

2. Salt the salad, season with mayonnaise, and garnish with green peas.

78.   SAUSAGE AND HAM SALAD

5 servings

Calorie content 1 serving - 100 kcal Cooking time - 10 min

INGREDIENTS

Cooked sausage - 200 g Ham - 100 g

Onions - 50 g

Pickled cucumbers - 200 g Vegetable oil - 20 ml Lemon juice - 10 ml Mustard - 0.5 tsp.

Salt and pepper to taste

PREPARATION METHOD

1. Peel the onions, cut into half rings and pour over boiling water to remove the bitterness.

2. Cut the sausage and ham into small pieces, combine with onions and chopped cucumbers.

3. To prepare dressing, mix vegetable oil, lemon juice, mustard, salt, and pepper. Pour the salad mixture with the mixture and put it in the refrigerator for 30 minutes

79.   SALAD GOOSE MEAT YUS APPLES

4 servings

Calorie content 1 serving - 190 kcal Cooking time - 30 min

INGREDIENTS

Boiled goose meat - 250 g Boiled potatoes - 250 g Apples - 200 g

Tomatoes - 100 g Lemon juice - 20 ml

Low-calorie mayonnaise - 150 g dill and parsley - 10 g salt to taste

PREPARATION METHOD

1. Peel potatoes from the skin and cut into cubes.

2. Peel the apples, remove the core, chop with a thin straw and sprinkle with lemon juice so that they do not darken

3. Cut the goose meat into small pieces.

4. Pour the tomatoes with boiling water, remove the peel, and cut the pulp into slices.

5. Put goose meat, apples, potatoes, tomatoes in a salad bowl, season the salad with mayonnaise, salt, mix, sprinkle with chopped greens dill and parsley and serve

80. CHICKEN AND CABBAGE SALAD

5 servings

Calorie content 1 serving - 70 kcal Cooking time - 15 min

<u>INGREDIENTS</u>

Boiled chicken meat - 300 g White cabbage - 300 g

Sour cream - 100 g Celery root - 20 g Boiled carrots - 50 g

Vegetable oil - 10 ml Grated horseradish - 5 g

Table vinegar - 5 ml Parsley - 10 g Sugar and salt to taste

PREPARATION METHOD

1. Chop cabbage.

2. Grate celery root

3. Cut the meat into strips or small cubes

4. Combine the prepared ingredients, add horseradish, vinegar, vegetable oil, salt, sugar, mix well and put in a slide in a salad bowl

5. Salad pours sour cream and garnish with sprigs of greens and mugs of carrots.

81. TURKEY AND APPLE SALAD

4 servings

Calorie content 1 serving - 110 kcal Cooking time - 20 min

INGREDIENTS

Boiled turkey meat - 250 g sweet apples - 200 g

Eggs - 2 pcs.

Pickled cucumber - 1 pc. Low-calorie mayonnaise - 100 g Lemon juice - 20 ml

Vinegar 3% - 20 ml

Ground black pepper and salt to taste.

<u>PREPARATION METHOD</u>

1. Cut the turkey meat into small pieces.

2. Peel and peel the apples, grate and sprinkle with lemon juice

3. Cut the cucumber into small cubes

4. Hard-boiled eggs, cool, peel, and grind.

5. To prepare dressing, combine mayonnaise, vinegar, salt and ground pepper

6. Put turkey meat, apples, cucumber, eggs in a salad bowl, pour dressing, mix and serve

82.   BOILED TONGUE SALAD

5 servings

Calorie content 1 serving - 100 kcal Cooking time - 40 min

<u>INGREDIENTS</u>

Boiled beef tongue - 300 g Low-calorie mayonnaise - 100 g Eggs - 4 pcs.

Carrots - 300 g Salted cucumbers - 200g Dill greens - 15 g Salt to taste

PREPARATION METHOD

1. Tongue cut into small pieces.

2. Boil the carrots, cool, peel, and chop.

3. Hard-boiled eggs, cool, peel and cut into slices.

4. Grind cucumbers and a part of green dill

5. Combine all ingredients, season with mayonnaise, salt, and mix

6. Put the finished salad in a salad bowl and decorate with sprigs of greens before serving.

83. CHICKEN BREAST SALAD WITH CANNED GREEN PEAS

4 servings

Calorie content 1 serving - 180 kcal Cooking time - 30 min

INGREDIENTS

Boiled chicken breast - 200 g Eggs - 2 pcs.

Boiled potatoes - 200 g Salted cucumbers - 150 g Soy mayonnaise - 200 g Onions - 50 g

Canned green peas - 100 g Boiled carrots - 2 pcs.

Dill and parsley - 10 g Salt to taste

PREPARATION METHOD

1. Cut the chicken breast into small pieces.

2. Hard-boiled eggs, cool, peel and grind

3. Cut the cucumbers into thin strips, carrots into slices, and potatoes into cubes.

4. Peel and chop onions

5. Wash parsley and dill and chop finely

6. Put the prepared ingredients in a salad bowl with canned green peas, salt, season with mayonnaise, mix and serve

84. ROAST DUCK SALAD

5 servings

Calorie content 1 serving - 150 kcal Cooking time - 20 min

INGREDIENTS

Roasted duck meat - 200 g Bacon - 150 g

Boiled white beans - 100 g Sour cream - 100 g

Low-calorie mayonnaise - 100 g Boiled eggs - 4 pcs.

Shredded dill greens - 15 g Parsley greens - 3 branches Salt to taste

PREPARATION METHOD

1. Cut the poultry meat and bacon into small pieces, 3 eggs into slices. Combine the prepared ingredients, add beans and dill, salt, season with sour cream and mayonnaise and mix gently.

2. Put the finished salad on a dish and decorate with parsley sprigs and slices of one egg before serving.

85. CHICKEN SALAD WITH APPLE AND TIERS

Calorie content 1 serving - 220 kcal Cooking time - 1 h 30 min

INGREDIENTS

Chicken - 800 g

Boiled rice - 30 g

Apple - 1 pc.

Carrots - 40 g

Green onion - 40 g Celery root - 40 g

Low-fat yogurt - 100 g Sour cream - 45 g

Vegetable oil - 1 tsp Melissa - 5 leaves Peppercorn pepper - 2 pcs.

Salt, ground white pepper, and saffron to taste.

PREPARATION METHOD

1. Bring water (2 L) to a boil, lower the washed chicken into it, bring to a boil again and remove the resulting foam.

2. Peel the carrots and celery root and add the foci to the bird along with peppercorns and salt. Boil until soft. Then remove the chicken from the broth, cool, remove the skin and bones and cut into small pieces.

3. To prepare the dressing, combine yogurt with sour cream, add oil, saffron, salt and pepper

4. Wash the apple, remove the core and cut into strips

5. Rice, chicken meat, apple, chopped carrots, green onions, cabbage celery, put in a salad bowl, pour dressing, mix

6. Before serving, sprinkle the salad with chopped lemon balm.

86. SALAD OF DUCK, CARROT, AND CURRANT

4 servings

Calorie content 1 serving - 180 kcal Cooking time - 20 min

INGREDIENTS

Boiled duck - 250 g Carrots - 450 g Red currants - 100 g Orange juice - 100 ml

Vegetable oil - 2 tbsp. Mint leaves - 4 pcs.

Sugar - 2 tsp

PREPARATION METHOD

1. Cut the boiled duck into small pieces

2. Peel, wash and grate the carrots on a coarse grater.

3. Put red currant berries and carrots in a salad bowl, sprinkle them with sugar, pour orange juice and vegetable oil, mix, lay the duck slices on top, mint leaves and put them on the table

87.   BEEF TONGUE SALAD WITH VEGETABLES

5 servings

Calorie content 1 serving - 50 kcal Cooking time - 30 min

INGREDIENTS

Boiled beef tongue - 300 g Low-calorie mayonnaise - 100 g Potatoes - 300 g

Yayla - 3-4 pcs. carrots - 200 g

Pickled Cucumbers - 200 g

Dill and parsley - 30 g Salt to taste

PREPARATION METHOD

1. Tongue cut into small pieces

2. Boil potatoes and carrots, cool, peel and cut into cubes.

3. Hard-boiled eggs, cool, peel and grind

4. Cucumbers mi dill and parsley finely chopped

5. Combine all ingredients, season with mayonnaise, salt, and mix well.

88.   MEAT SALAD

5 servings

Calorie content 1 serving - 60 kcal Cooking time - 15 min

INGREDIENTS

Boiled veal - 300 g Pickled mushrooms - 100 g Low-calorie mayonnaise - 100 g Boiled potatoes - 200g, Eggs - 2 pcs.

Salted cucumber - 100 g Parsley - 10 g Mustard - 5g. Salt and pepper to taste

PREPARATION METHOD

1. Cut boiled meat into slices.

2. Hard-boiled eggs, cool, peel, and chop

3. Cut the potatoes into cubes, cucumber, and mushrooms - in strips

4. Combine, salt, pepper, season with mayonnaise mixed with mustard

5. Before serving, decorate the salad with chopped parsley.

89.   BEEF AND CANNED GREEN PEAS SALAD

4 servings

Calorie content with 1 serving - 200 kcal. Cooking time - 40 min

INGREDIENTS

Boiled beef - 200 g Potatoes - 3 pcs.

Pickled cucumbers - 2 pcs. Eggs - 3 pcs.

Canned green peas - 100 g Dill and parsley - 10 g

Low-calorie mayonnaise - 250 g Salt to taste

PREPARATION METHOD

1. Cook potatoes in their skins, cool, peel, and cut into cubes.

2. Chop pickles.

3. Cut the beef into small pieces

4. Hard-boiled eggs, cool, peel and grind

5. Wash dill and parsley, dry, and chop finely.

6. Put the prepared ingredients in a salad bowl with canned green peas, salt to taste, season with mayonnaise, mix and serve

90. BOILED HAM SALAD WILLOW CAULIFLOWER

4 servings

Calorie content 1 serving - 150 kcal Cooking time - 40 min

INGREDIENTS

Boiled ham - 200 g Boiled turnip - 200 g Boiled carrots - 2 pcs. Cauliflower - 120 g

Canned green peas - 70 g Low-calorie mayonnaise - 100 g

Dill and parsley - 10 g Salt to taste

PREPARATION METHOD

1. Cut the ham into strips

2. Peel and cut carrots and turnips into small pieces

3. Boil cauliflower inflorescences in salted water for 10 minutes, then cool and grind.

4. Put prepared ingredients in a salad bowl together with canned green peas, pour with mayonnaise, mix and serve, sprinkled with finely chopped parsley or dill

91. BEEF AND TOMATO SALAD

5 servings

Calorie content 1 serving - 80 kcal Cooking time - 15 min

INGREDIENTS

Boiled lean beef - 200 g Tomatoes - 500 g

Fresh cucumbers - 200 g Onions - 100 g

Sour cream - 200 g Pepper and salt to taste

PREPARATION METHOD

1. Cut the meat into strips.

2. Wash and chop tomatoes.

3. Peel the cucumbers and cut into circles

4. Chop the onion finely

5. Mix all ingredients, pepper, salt, and season with sour cream.

6. Before serving, decorate the salad with slices of tomato and slices of cucumber.

92. SALAD WITH CHEESE AND HAM

4 servings

Calorie content 1 serving - 225 kcal. Cooking time - 20 min

INGREDIENTS

Smoked ham - 150 g Cheddar cheese - 150 g Sweet pepper - 1 pc.

Celery Greens - 10 g

Greens and parsley - 10 g Leaf lettuce - 50 g Soy mayonnaise - 3 tbsp.

Vegetable oil - 1 tbsp. Wine vinegar - 1 tbsp.

Salt to taste

PREPARATION METHOD

1. Cut the cheddar cheese into small cubes

2. Wash sweet peppers, cut in half, remove seeds and chop the pulp

3. Cut the ham into small pieces.

4. Wash the herbs of the tarpaulin, parsley, celery, and chop

5. Lettuce leaves break into small pieces.

6. Put the prepared ingredients in a salad bowl, salt to taste, season with a mixture made from vegetable oil, mayonnaise whose vinegar, mix and serve

93. VEAL SALAD WITH CAULIFLOWER

5 servings

Calorie content 1 serving - 170 kcal Cooking time - 30 min

INGREDIENTS

Boiled veal - 200 g Potatoes - 150 g Cauliflower - 100 g

Canned green peas - 100 g Cucumbers - 2 pcs.

Tomatoes - 2 pcs.

Apples - 100 g. Eggs - 2 pcs. Low-calorie mayonnaise - 200 g Leaf lettuce - 100 g

Parsley - 10 g Sable to taste

<u>PREPARATION METHOD</u>

1. Diced boiled veal

2. Peel the apples, remove the core and chop.

3. Hard-boiled eggs, cool, peel and cut into slices.

4. Cook the potatoes. uniform and cut into cubes.

5. Wash cauliflower, sort into inflorescences, boil in salted water, cool and grind.

6. Pour the tomatoes with boiling water, peel and cut into slices, cucumbers in half circles, salad in thin strips

7. Wash and chop the parsley

8. Put the prepared ingredients in a salad bowl with canned peas, season with mayonnaise, mix, and serve.

94. CHICKEN SALAD WITH RED CABBAGE

5 servings

Caloric content of the 1st serving - 65 kcal. Cooking time - 20 min

<u>INGREDIENTS</u>

Fried chicken fillet - 300 g Red cabbage - 200 g Apple - 1 pc.

Canned corn - 30 g Olive oil - 20 ml

Lemon juice - 10 ml Sugar - 5 g

Parsley - 10 g pain and pepper to taste

PREPARATION METHOD

1. Wash the cabbage, chop, salt and mix with chopped chicken meat.

2. Put the ingredients in a slide on a flat dish, garnish with sliced apple and corn

3. Mix olive oil with lemon juice, sugar, salt, and pepper, pour the salad over the resulting sauce, and let it brew for 30 minutes. Then sprinkle the dish with chopped parsley and fall on the table.

95. SALAD WITH SAUSAGE AND CANNED GREEN PEAS

5 servings

Calorie content 1 serving - 100 kcal cooking time - 30 min

INGREDIENTS

Cooked sausage - 300 g

Low-calorie mayonnaise - 200 g

Canned green peas - 150 g pickles - 400 g

Potatoes - 250 g Carrots – 200g

Dill and parsley - 10 g Salt and pepper to taste

PREPARATION METHOD

1. Boil potatoes and carrots in salted water, cool, peel and cut into strips

2. Cucumbers peel it. chop

3. Dice sausage

4. Combine all ingredients, add green peas, salt, pepper, season with mayonnaise, and mix thoroughly.

5. Ready salad before serving garnish with chopped herbs.

96.   CHICKEN AND FRUIT SALAD

4 servings

Calorie content 1 serving - 140 kcal Cooking time - 30 min

INGREDIENTS

Boiled chicken meat - 200 g

Seedless grapes - 150 g Oranges - 200 g

Sweet apples - 150 g Egg - 1 pc.

Low-calorie mayonnaise - 120 g Lemon juice - 10 ml

Sugar - 20 g

Ground black pepper and salt to taste.

<u>PREPARATION METHOD</u>

1. Hard-boiled egg, cool, peel and grind

2. Chicken meat into small pieces

3. Wash and cut the grapes in half each berry

4. Peel the oranges from the peel and internal partitions and cut the pulp into small pieces.

5. Apple peel and core and chop

6. To prepare the dressing, combine mayonnaise with lemon juice, sugar, salt, pepper, and mix.

7. Put chicken meat, egg, apples, grapes, and oranges in a salad bowl, pour dressing and serve

97. BEEF TENDERLOIN AND RADISH SALAD

2 servings

Calorie content 1 serving - 180 kcal Cooking time - 30 min

INGREDIENTS

Beef tenderloin - 100 g Cucumber - 1 pc.

Radish - 35 g Cognac - 20 ml

Vegetable oil - 30 ml Mustard, salt and pepper to taste

PREPARATION METHOD

1. Wash and chop radishes.

2. Peel the cucumber and cut into strips

3. Prepare the prepared ingredients with mustard, salt, and pepper.

4. Cut the beef tenderloin into thin slices, fry in vegetable oil until browning, add salad dressing, sprinkle with cognac, and serve the table.

98. CHICKEN SALAD

5 servings

Calorie content 1 serving - 55 kcal Cooking time - 15 min

INGREDIENTS

Boiled chicken meat - 200 g Celery roots - 10 pcs.

Low-calorie mayonnaise - 5 tbsp. Lemon - 1 pc.

Salt and pepper to taste

PREPARATION METHOD

1. Peel the celery roots, cut into strips and sprinkle with freshly squeezed lemon juice, then grind with salt until soft

2. Cut the chicken meat into small cubes, then mix the prepared ingredients.

3. Salad season with mayonnaise, add salt and pepper

99.   HAM AND MEAT SALAD

5 servings

Calorie content of 1 portion - 112 kcal

Cooking time - 30 min.

INGREDIENTS

Boiled meat - 200 g Beef ham - 100 g Boiled tongue - 100 g Pickled cucumbers - 100 g Egg - 1 pc.

Sour cream - 50 g

Parsley - 10 g Salt to the floor to taste

PREPARATION METHOD

1. Cut the meat, ham, and tongue into small pieces

2. Hard-boiled egg, cool, peel and grind

3. Peel the cucumbers and cut into cubes.

4. Combine all the ingredients, salt, season with sour cream, mix well, and put in a salad bowl.

5. Before serving, decorate the salad with chopped greens.

100. BOILED HAM AND GRAPE SALAD

5 servings

Calorie content 1 serving - 160 kcal Cooking time - 20 min

INGREDIENTS

Cooked ham - 120 g Seedless grapes - 500 g Hard cheese - 120 g

Apples - 100 g

Chopped almonds - 120 g

Low-calorie mayonnaise - 3 tbsp. Sour milk - 120 ml

Lemon juice - 10 ml

Ground black pepper powder to taste

PREPARATION METHOD

1. Cheese cut into small cubes

2. Peel the apples Asht the peel and core, chop the pulp and sprinkle with lemon juice.

3. Cut the ham into small pieces.

4. Berries of grapes cut in half

5. Put the prepared ingredients in a salad bowl with almonds and pour dressing made from mayonnaise, sour milk, salt, and pepper.

6. Mix the salad and serve the henna table.

101. EGG FILLET CHICKEN SALAD WITH EGGS

5 servings

Calorie content 1 serving - 95 kcal Cooking time - 30 min

INGREDIENTS

Chicken fillet - 300 g

Canned green peas - 50 g Low-calorie mayonnaise - 50 g

Pickled cucumbers - 300 g Boiled potatoes - 200 g Boiled carrots - 200 g Olive oil - 20 g

Boiled eggs - 2-3 pcs.

Cilantro Greens - 15 g Salt to taste

PREPARATION METHOD

1. Finely chop the meat, fry in oil, cool and combine with chopped cucumbers, potatoes and carrots, chopped eggs and chopped green cheese.

2. Salt the salad, season with mayonnaise and serve, garnished with green peas.

102. LIVER SALAD

5 servings

Calorie content 1 serving - 80 kcal Cooking time - 40 min

INGREDIENTS

Beef liver - 300g

Dark seedless grapes - 100 g Onions - 200 g

Carrots - 200 g Leaf lettuce - 20 g Butter - 20 g

Vegetable oil - 20 ml

Salt, red and black pepper powder to taste

PREPARATION METHOD

1. Rinse the liver, cut into small pieces, and stew it in a pan in a small amount of water. Then cool, pepper and salt.

2. Peel the onions and carrots and cut into strips, then fry them in butter, add the liver to them and simmer them on low heat for 4-5 minutes

3. Wash the grapes, cut each berry in half

4. Combine all the ingredients, salt to taste, season with vegetable oil and mix gently.

5. Put the finished salad in a salad bowl and garnish with chopped stripes before serving lettuce leaves.

103. BOILED VEAL SALAD WITH GREEN PEAS

5 servings

Calorie content 1 serving - 108 kcal Cooking time - 15 min

<u>INGREDIENTS</u>

Boiled veal - 400 g Low-calorie mayonnaise - 100 g

Canned green peas - 20 g Boiled egg - 1 pc.

Garlic - 30 g

Basil greens - 20 g Salt and pepper to taste

<u>PREPARATION METHOD</u>

1. Dice the meat, add peeled and chopped garlic, finely chopped basil greens, mayonnaise, salt and pepper

2. Mix everything, put in a slide on a dish, garnish with green peas and peeled and sliced egg.

104. GREEN SALAD WITH CHICKEN AND EGGS

4 servings

Calorie content 1 serving - 160 kcal Cooking time - 20 min

<u>INGREDIENTS</u>

Leaf lettuce - 300 g Eggs - 2 pcs.

Boiled Chicken - 200 g

Sour cream - 125 g Vinegar 3% - 1 tsp

Dill Ai parsley - 10 g

Ground black pepper and salt to taste.

PREPARATION METHOD

1. Hard-boiled eggs, cool, peel and cut into slices.

2. Wash, dry and lettuce leaves into small pieces

3. Finely chop the chicken

4. Wash dill and parsley

5. To prepare the dressing, mix sour cream with salt, ground black pepper and vinegar, and mix thoroughly

6. Put chicken, eggs, leaf lettuce, parsley or dill in a salad bowl, pour sour cream and seek on the table

105. CHICKEN SALAD WITH JAAPELSIN CHEESE

5 servings

Calorie content 1 serving - 55 kcal Cooking time - 15 min

INGREDIENTS

Fried chicken fillet - 200 g Grated cheese - 100 g

Apple - 1 pc. Orange - 1 pc.

Low-calorie mayonnaise - 50 g Lhuk green, salt, and pepper to taste.

<u>PREPARATION METHOD</u>

1. Chop the chicken fillet

2. Peel the orange, divide into slices, then cut into cubes

3. Chop the apple by first removing the core

4. Mix all ingredients, put in a shallow container, salt, pepper, season with mayonnaise.

5. Put the finished dish in a salad bowl, sprinkle with grated cheese, chopped green onions and drive up to the table

106. CHICKEN SALAD WITH GREEN PEAS AND EGGS

5 servings

Calorie content of 1 portion - 100 kcal. Cooking time - 15 min

<u>INGREDIENTS</u>

Roasted Chicken Meat - 200 g Ham - 150 g

Canned green peas - 100 g Sour cream - 50 g

Low-calorie mayonnaise - 50 g Eggs - 4 pcs.

Shredded ukrodpa - 20 g Parsley - 5 g

Salt and pepper to taste

PREPARATION METHOD

1. Cut the poultry meat and ham into small pieces.

2. Hard-boiled eggs, cool, peel, and chop (leave one egg for decoration)

3. Combine the prepared ingredients, add peas and dill to them, salt, pepper, season with sour cream and mayonnaise and mix gently

4. Before serving, decorate the finished salad with sprigs of parsley and slices of one egg.

107. SAUSAGE SALAD WITH PICKLED CUCUMBERS

5 servings

Calorie content 1 serving - 180 kcal Cooking time - 30 min

INGREDIENTS

Cooked sausage - 200 g Smoked sausage - 100 g Ham - 100 g

Onion peeling - 100 g Pickled cucumbers - 300 g Vegetable oil - 20 ml Lemon juice - 10 ml Mustard - 0.5 tsp.

Salt and pepper to taste

<u>PREPARATION METHOD</u>

1. Peel onions, cut into half rings and pour over boiling water to remove the bitterness

2. Cut the sausage, ham, and cucumbers into small pieces and combine with onion

3. To prepare the dressing, mix vegetable oil, lemon juice, mustard, salt, chi pepper.

Pour the salad into it or put it in the refrigerator for 30 minutes.

108. SALAD OF FRIED CHICKEN AND FRESH CUCUMBERS

4 servings

Calorie content 1 serving - 200 kcal Cooking time - 30 min

<u>INGREDIENTS</u>

Fried chicken - 200 g Boiled potato - 150 g Cucumbers - 2 pcs.

Leaf lettuce - 40 g Eggs - 3 pcs.

Canned green peas - 50 g Low-calorie mayonnaise - 200g

Dill Greens - 10 g Salt to taste

PREPARATION METHOD

1. Hard-boiled eggs, cool, peel and grind

2. Cut the potatoes into cubes, and the chicken - in small pieces.

3. Wash lettuce leaves, dry, and cut into thin strips.

4. Peel the cucumbers and chop.

5. Prepared ingredients will be laid out in a junkyard along with canned green peas, salt, add mayonnaise, mix and put on the table, garnished with finely chopped dill.

CONCLUSION

Maintaining a healthy and balanced diet is not an easy task, especially for those who are not focused or have the willpower. A good tip for anyone who wants to switch from an unhealthy caloric diet to a nutritious and healthy diet is to study well the types of foods such as their vitamins, their calories, etc. Knowing foods well can form or create a healthy diet plan with foods that are pleasing to the taste of each person.

The Mediterranean diet is very rich in many ways, besides being based on regular physical activity, which does not necessarily force the adept to go to a gym, but a walk is enough, it has many benefits, besides being rich in Antioxidant foods and good fats like olive oil are rich in fruits, vegetables, legumes, cereals, almonds and walnuts, foods that help increase metabolism and prevent heart disease.

There are numerous studies done on the Mediterranean diet, and many prove its effectiveness. Several studies have shown a decrease in bad cholesterol and an increase in good cholesterol, as well as a gradual decrease in weight and abdominal fat.

The Mediterranean diet is highly recommended by many nutritionists because of the many benefits it has; however, it is a proven fact that this diet has a disadvantage that has to be taken into consideration: the Mediterranean diet is considered expensive because it consumes preferentially. fish such as tuna, salmon, tilapia, in addition to the daily consumption of nuts and nuts, many fruits and vegetables. However, it can, of course, fit into everyone's pocket, but it will have its benefits reduced compared to the person who eats according to the original rules.

The Mediterranean diet must be tailored to your specifications, and your success is guaranteed if you strictly follow it. Have a food routine, avoid fatty and calorie foods, always have a fruit and cereal bar to feel that hunger between meals will help you successfully complete your goals.

Having a healthy and balanced diet is a fundamental part for those who want to stay healthy, young, and beautiful. It is not just a matter of being fit, but a long-term investment for your health and well being. The fit body is a consequence of a healthy and balanced lifestyle and is welcome to each of us.